D1595270

Interventional Treatment of Advanced Ischemic Heart Disease

Reynolds Delgado   *Editor*

Harvinder Singh Arora   *Associate Editor*

Interventional Treatment of Advanced Ischemic Heart Disease

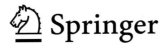 Springer

Editor

Reynolds Delgado
Texas Heart Institute
Houston, TX 77225-0345
USA

Associate Editor

Harvinder Singh Arora
Texas Heart Institute
Houston, TX 77225-0345
USA

ISBN 978-1-84800-394-1   e-ISBN 978-1-84800-395-8
DOI 10.1007/978-1-84800-395-8

British Library Cataloguing in Publication Data
A catalogue record for this book is available from the British Library

Library of Congress Control Number: 2008942075

© Springer-Verlag London Limited 2009
Apart from any fair dealing for the purposes of research or private study, or criticism or review, as permitted under the Copyright, Designs and Patents Act 1988, this publication may only be reproduced, stored or transmitted, in any form or by any means, with the prior permission in writing of the publishers, or in the case of reprographic reproduction in accordance with the terms of licenses issued by the Copyright Licensing Agency. Enquiries concerning reproduction outside those terms should be sent to the publishers.
The use of registered names, trademarks, etc., in this publication does not imply, even in the absence of a specific statement, that such names are exempt from the relevant laws and regulations and therefore free for general use.
Product liability: The publisher can give no guarantee for information about drug dosage and application thereof contained in this book. In every individual case the respective user must check its accuracy by consulting other pharmaceutical literature.

Printed on acid-free paper

Springer Science+Business Media
springer.com

In Memoriam

Branislav ("Brano") Radovancevic, a legend in the international heart-failure community. Born in Osijek , Croatia , Brano completed his medical degree in Belgrade, Serbia. In 1984, he joined the Cardiopulmonary Transplantation Department of the Texas Heart Institute (THI) at St. Luke's Episcopal Hospital, as research fellow. He quickly became an invaluable member of the transplant program. As an emerging leader in immunosuppression, immunology, and transplant research, Brano was highly respected nationally and internationally. His early research into therapies to prevent and manage organ rejection was recognized worldwide.

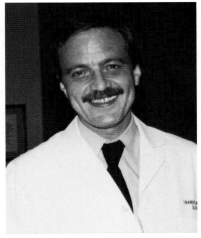

Owing to his tireless efforts, Brano became Associate Director of Transplant Research in 1998 and Director of the Center for Cardiac Support in 2005. In the latter capacity, he lectured and traveled extensively, sharing his knowledge and expertise about mechanical circulatory support, heart transplantation, and other heart failure therapies with colleagues and friends.

As an integral member of THI's animal research team, Brano designed and preformed studies involving myocardial protection during cardiac operations, as well as temporary and permanent mechanical circulatory assist devices, heart valve prostheses, and synthetic vascular grafts. In addition he authored, and co- authored approximately 300 publications, and oversaw the writing of numerous heart failure and transplant protocols.

For the annual THI symposium, he developed and hosted the famous "Rodeo Meeting," bringing top cardiologists and surgeons from around the country to debate topics in transplantation. Introduced in 1994, the Rodeo Meeting still exists, having grown steadily throughout the years.

Until his death in September 2007, Brano continued to make invaluable contributions to the field of heart transplantation, particularly immunosuppression of the transplant patient, and to other areas of cardiovascular research. His commitment to the fight against heart disease and his compassion for his patients helped make THI an unparalleled bastion of cardiovascular research. Indeed Brano exemplified the mission Dr. Denton A. Cooley envisioned in 1962, when he founded THI: to reduce the devastating toll of cardiovascular disease through innovative programs in research, education, and improved patient care. Although Brano is no longer physically present, his legacy will continue to inspire his medical colleagues and to benefit heart failure patients everywhere.

Preface

The problem of ischemic heart disease is one of the most important public health problems in the world today. With more effective treatment for acute coronary syndromes and the aging of the population, more people are now living with coronary artery disease and advanced ischemic heart disease is becoming increasingly prevalent. Heart failure is the final endpoint for patients who survive myocardial infarctions and sudden cardiac death, and now ischemic heart disease accounts for greater than 60% of heart failure cases. The toll in death and suffering of ischemic heart failure is enormous with cardiovascular disease as the number one killer and a lifetime risk of developing heart failure of one in five in both men and women. Chronic heart failure and coronary disease is a cost that is fast becoming overwhelming for the health care system in the United States and other countries and costs are only increasing. It is because of these facts that we have sought to create a text that will specifically address the problem of advanced ischemic heart disease.

Many believe that advanced ischemic heart disease will soon become the most challenging clinical problem facing the cardiovascular physician. It is ironic that this problem is the result of the successes of medicine to date in lengthening lifespan and treating acute myocardial infarction. There has been a tremendous improvement in survival from heart attack and with this has come more heart failure. In addition, heart failure patients are living longer due to advances in medical therapy, adding to the problem. Certainly, understanding of risk factors and their modification has decreased the incidence of stroke and heart attack but as those patients survive, many develop heart failure due to the inexorable progression of coronary artery disease.

Rather than focusing on a specific disease state such as coronary artery disease or heart failure in this text, we sought to focus on the concept of the patient with advanced ischemic heart disease as embodied in the discussion above. As such we define advanced ischemic heart disease for the purposes of this text as disease of the heart caused by coronary atherosclerosis which results in significant heart failure signs and symptoms or intractable angina and thus severely limits lifestyle or longevity. There have been volumes written on the diagnosis and treatment of coronary artery disease and heart failure. The treatment of these has now been standardized to the point that there are very well established guidelines promulgated by the American Heart Association and The American College of Cardiology. This text will strive to pick up where the guidelines leave off and address the real challenge of patients with advanced ischemic heart disease. Many have the bias that once severe heart failure has occurred due to coronary artery disease that there is little to offer in the therapeutic realm. Though therapy is clearly challenging, new advances are making effective therapy of these patients truly possible. This text embodies that notion. Finally, there is much still to learn about the basic mechanisms of the progression of heart failure due to coronary artery disease and how best to assess these therapeutic options. The text will address these with a focus on treatment so that it may be a practical reference for the practicing clinician and well as the basic or clinical researcher and student.

The text will begin with a discussion of the problem and its effect on society and the practicing cardiovascular physician. It will then explore the basic mechanisms by which advanced ischemic heart disease develops after initial myocardial infarction. This is an area which is of profound importance if this growing problem is to be adequately addressed. Prevention of heart failure after initial heart attack is also very important and will be addressed next, followed by a critical discussion of the controversy and methods of determining viability in making decisions about revascularization. Heart failure due to ischemic heart disease then will be studied followed by its treatment. In these sections, we explore those things perhaps not easily found in the guidelines with these complicated patients with multiple comorbid conditions. Angina, though less common with modern medical therapy and revascularization techniques is still a major limitation to a quality lifestyle in these patients and will be discussed. Sudden cardiac death is still the most common mode of death and modern implantable defibrillator therapy holds the potential for great benefit and will be discussed in Chapter 8. Cardiac resynchronization therapy is an important new technology which is currently being refined and will be discussed next.

Much study has gone into the two major modes of revascularization, percutaneous and surgical and this has historically focused on the patient with preserved systolic function, we will address this in light of the patient with heart failure, a complex topic and one of timely importance with advances in stent technology and surgical technique. Mitral valve and left ventricular remodeling surgery have been sources of great interest and controversy and will be addressed next. Following this, we will explore mechanical assist and replacement device therapy which is of great interest as it is clear that this, in its various forms will play a dominant role in the future. The possibility of device therapy to supplant need for transplant now and in the future will then be discussed. Transplant is still an outstanding therapy for eligible patients but is severely limited by donor shortage. Finally, the future is bright and new technologies such as a completely implanted total artificial heart and cellular implantation therapies exemplify this. Beyond this, new advances in understanding genomics and proteinomics are leading to scientific advances which hold great promise. These and other exciting new therapies will be explored in the final chapter.

Advanced ischemic heart disease is fast becoming one of the most challenging problems facing the modern cardiovascular physician and current established therapies often fail to adequately address this population of patients. As therapy of heart disease evolves, we need to address the challenging questions posed by this clinical problem. We hope that *Interventional Treatment of Advanced Ischemic Heart Disease* will aid you in the study and treatment of these patients who deserve the best that modern medicine can provide them.

Houston, Texas   Reynolds Delgado
USA   Harvinder Singh Arora

Contents

Contributors

Harvinder Singh Arora, MD, MPH Texas Heart Institute, St. Luke's Episcopal Hospital, Houston, TX, USA

Nitish Badhwar, MD Department of Medicine, University of California, San Francisco, CA, USA

Marianne Bergheim Texas Heart Institute, St. Luke's Episcopal Hospital, Houston, TX, USA

John P. Boehmer, MD Division of Cardiology, The Heart and Vascular Institute, The Penn State Hershey Medical Center, The Pennsylvania State University College of Medicine, Hershey, PA 17033, USA

Reynolds Delgado, MD Texas Heart Institute, St. Luke's Episcopal Hospital, Houston, TX, USA

James J. Ferguson, MD Department of Surgical and Critical Care, The Medicines Company, Parsippany, NJ, USA; Baylor College of Medicine, Texas Heart Institute at St. Luke's Episcopal Hospital, Houston, TX, USA

Gregory M. Giesler, MD Division of Cardiology, University of Texas Health Science Center, Memorial Hermann Hospital, Houston, TX, USA

K. Lance Gould, MD Division of Cardiology, University of Texas Health Science Center at Houston, Houston, TX, USA

John L. Jefferies, MD Texas Heart Institute, St. Luke's Episcopal Hospital, Houston, TX, USA

Catalin Loghin, MD Division of Cardiology, University of Texas Health Science Center, Houston, Houston, TX, USA

Teresa De Marco, MD Cardiac Electrophysiology Section, Department of Medicine, University of California, San Francisco, CA, USA

Dipsu Patel, MD The University of Texas Health Science Center, Houston, TX, USA

Emerson C. Perin, MD, PhD Stem Cell Center, Texas Heart Institute, St. Luke's Episcopal Hospital, Houston, TX, USA

Guilherme V. Silva, MD Stem Cell Center, Texas Heart Institute, St. Luke's Episcopal Hospital, Houston, TX, USA

Richard W. Smalling, MD, PhD Department of Internal Medicine-Cardiology, University of Texas, Medical School Houston, Houston, TX, USA

Zian H. Tseng, MD, MAS Cardiac Electrophysiology Section, Department of Medicine, University of California, San Francisco, CA, USA

James T. Willerson, MD Texas Heart Institute, St. Luke's Episcopal Hospital, Houston, TX, USA

Chapter 1
The Problems of Advanced Ischemic Heart Disease

Epidemiology, Growth Rate, Burden, and Costs of AIHD

James J. Ferguson and Dipsu Patel

Introduction

Houston, we've had a problem

With these words, on April 13, 1970 the Apollo XIII astronauts notified Mission Control in Houston that a devastating explosion had taken place in Service Module oxygen tank #2. The three astronauts, James A. Lovell, Jr., Fred W. Haise, Jr., and John L. Swigert, Jr., were thousands of miles from Earth, headed in the wrong direction, and their lives were in imminent danger. What followed was a heroic tale of ingenuity, resourcefulness, courage, and dedication as the three astronauts abandoned the command module, continued their voyage around the moon, and returned successfully to earth on April 17, 1970. Hollywood drama aside, this was not a matter of pulling rabbits out of a magical engineering hat, it was the result of thousands of hours of training, simulation, preparation, and anticipation [1].

Western society is currently facing a public health crisis of astounding proportions, but this has not come in the form of a sudden explosion, and there are a lot more than three lives at risk. The problem of advanced ischemic heart disease (AIHD) has been with us throughout history, but we are now confronting a veritable epidemic of the disease, and are only now beginning to recognize how pervasive the problem is, how rapidly it is growing (and will continue to grow in the immediate future), and the burden that it imposes on our health care system and society as a whole. With our ever-expanding therapeutic options, the problem only multiplies as our medical advances allow extended survival of these patients.

Houston, we have a *real* problem, and a problem that only gets worse as our treatments get better.

Unfortunately, there is no magical cardiovascular mission control that we can appeal to, to guide us in the management of this problem, and bring us safely back to earth. Yes, there are thousands of dedicated scientists, and health professionals working in the background, but this problem is not one that can be "fixed" and "go away," this problem is going to be part of all of our lives and, in all likelihood, an even bigger part of our children's lives. We, as physicians, scientists, and health professionals, are going to be in the front lines of a battle, a battle we cannot hope to actually "win" in the foreseeable future, but one in which our goal is to minimize the casualties in our patients and to society. The only way to fight such a battle is to be armed, not only with an assortment of diagnostic and therapeutic weaponry, but, more importantly to be armed with *information* about the enemy of AIHD. By truly understanding the scope of the problem we can best direct our diagnostic (reconnaissance) and therapeutic (strategic and tactical) approaches to improving the outcome of our patients.

This initial chapter sets the stage for what is to come in subsequent chapters on the diagnostic and therapeutic approaches to AIHD and the consequences faced by these patients. The present chapter

J.J. Ferguson (✉)
Baylor College of Medicine, Texas Heart Institute, St. Luke's Episcopal Hospital, Houston, TX, USA

R. Delgado, H.S. Arora (eds.), *Interventional Treatment of Advanced Ischemic Heart Disease*,
DOI 10.1007/978-1-84800-395-8_1, © Springer-Verlag London Limited 2009

describes the prevalence, the growth rate, and the clinical and societal consequences of AIHD. As Dr. Delgado and Dr. Radovancevic noted in the preface, there are more people currently living with AIHD than ever before. Cardiovascular disease is the leading cause of mortality worldwide, and the consequences will progress to the severe advance of heart failure in one out of five men and women.

Yes, Houston, we have a problem, but giving up, surrendering, is not an option. The first step in our battle against AIHD and its sequellae is to understand as much of the enemy as possible.

Epidemiology

It is estimated that there are more than 70,000,000 patients in the United States with one or more types of cardiovascular disease [2]. This includes more than 65,000,000 with hypertension, 13,000,000 with coronary heart disease, approximately 4,900,000 with congestive heart failure, and 5,400,000 with stroke. Of the patients with coronary heart disease, there are approximately 7,100,000 who have had a myocardial infarction (MI) and 6,400,000 who have angina pectoris. Approximately 300,000–900,000 of these angina patients have refractory symptoms, a number that is growing at the rate of 25,000–75,000 cases per year [3].Worldwide, it is estimated that cardiovascular disease accounts for about one out of every three deaths [4].

In the United States, one of every four individuals has some form of cardiovascular disease; these numbers are growing daily, particularly as the age distribution of our population becomes increasingly skewed toward the higher end. The Framingham study has documented that the rate of new first cardiovascular events rises dramatically with age, from 7/1,000 in men aged 35–44 to 35–44/1,000 in men aged 85–94 [5]. Men under the age of 75 have a higher proportion of cardiovascular events due to ischemic coronary heart disease, while women have a higher proportion of events attributable to CHF. In American women there is about one death per minute caused by cardiovascular disease. This translates into more than 500,000 deaths per year in women, or more than the next six most frequent causes of death put together.

Moreover, aging of our population will be even more of a problem in the coming decades. By 2010 it is estimated that there will be 40,000,000 men and women with coronary heart disease.

In the overall US population, cardiovascular disease claims one life every 34 s, or more than the next five most frequent causes of death put together (cancer, chronic lower pulmonary disease, accidents, diabetes, and influenza and pneumonia). In 2002 cardiovascular disease accounted for 38% of all morbid events in the United States—1 of every 2.6 deaths (Figs. 1.1 and 1.2) [6]. It is estimated that approximately half a million people die of heart disease either before reaching the hospital or in the emergency department.

Focusing more closely on CAD, in 2002 an estimated 13 million Americans had coronary artery disease, 7.1 million had a history of MI; there were 865,000 new MIs that year, with approximately 500,000 deaths, and 2.1 million hospital discharges. It is currently estimated that approximately half a million people will have a recurrent MI and there will be approximately 175,000 new silent MIs noted incidentally. In people aged 40–74, the prevalence of MI is higher in men, but the prevalence of angina is higher in women [7]. Thus, while men die more frequently, there may be more women alive with the disease. The rate of CAD in women increases substantially (two- to threefold) after menopause (Figs. 1.3 and 1.4) [9]. The average age for a first MI is approximately 66 years in men and 70 years in women. More than one half of all cardiovascular events in men and women under the age of 75 are attributable to CAD. In fact, CAD is the single leading cause of death in men and women, producing one new coronary event every 26 s, and one new death every minute. The mortality of people who have an event is more than 40% [7]. Figure 1.5 shows the US age-adjusted death rates for heart disease by age and gender [10].

And while the data on coronary artery disease are sobering, in many ways they merely represent the tip of the iceberg when considering the prevalence of risk factors for coronary artery disease (Fig. 1.6). Obesity and diabetes are approaching epidemic proportions (Fig. 1.7). Seven out of every ten American adults are considered overweight (BMI ≥ 25) and three out of ten are obese (BMI ≥ 30) [7]. The prevalence of obesity has increased 75%

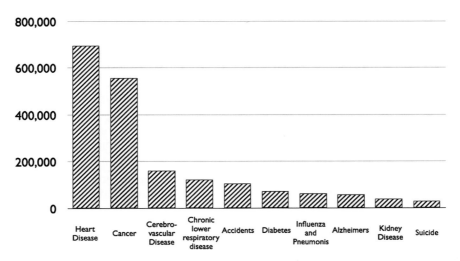

Fig. 1.1 Leading causes of death in US, 2002. Adapted from reference [6]

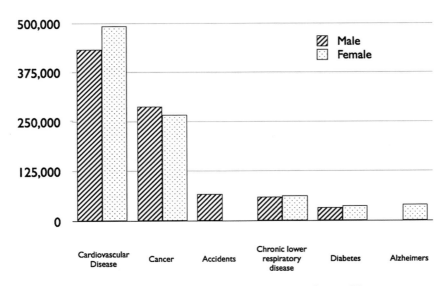

Fig. 1.2 Leading causes of death—US men and women, 2002. Adapted from reference [2]

over the last 15 years, across all ethnic groups (Fig. 1.8) [11–15]. A recent study in 1,740 eighth graders (mean age 13.6 ± 0.6 years) documented a mean BMI of 24.3 ± 5.9 [16].

In parallel, the prevalence of diabetes has increased by 61% in the last 15 years (Fig. 1.9) [13–15]. In 2002 there were approximately 13.9 million Americans (6.7% of the population) with a

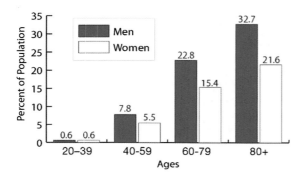

Fig. 1.3 Prevalence of coronary heart disease by age and sex, NHANES (1999–2002). Adapted from reference [8]

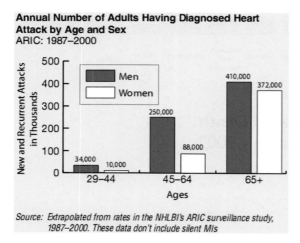

Fig. 1.4 The US incidence of MI by age and sex. Adapted from reference [8]

diagnosis of diabetes, an estimated 5.9 million (2.8% of the population) with undiagnosed diabetes, and 14.5% million (7% of the population) with pre-diabetes. In that same survey of eighth graders noted earlier [16], 40.5% had a fasting glucose ≥100 mg/dL (impaired fasting glucose) and 2% had a 2-h post-prandial glucose of > 140 mg/dL (impaired glucose tolerance). About 70% of patients with diabetes die as a consequence of cardiovascular disease. The death rate in diabetic adults is 2–4 times higher in diabetics than in nondiabetics (Fig. 1.10) [17]. Diabetes also provides substantial additive risk in the presence of other risk factors (Table 1.1).

Hypertension and hypercholesterolemia are also on the rise [18]. An estimated 65 million Americans

(almost one third of the US population) had hypertension in 2002 and there are probably close to 60 million Americans who have "pre-hypertension." Of those with hypertension, almost one third are unaware of it, and one fourth may be treated but inadequately controlled. Hypertension is present in about one half of people with a first heart attack. A history of hypertension is also present in more than 90% of patients who develop congestive heart failure and increase the risk of developing CHF two- to threefold.

In 2002, 50.7% of the US population had a total cholesterol > 200 mg/dL, 18.3% had a total cholesterol > 240 mg/dL, 45.8% had an LDL cholesterol > 130 mg/dL, and 26.4% had an HDL cholesterol < 40 mg/dL. Of the people who would otherwise qualify for lipid-lowering therapy, less than half of them are actually receiving any form of treatment [9]. In the US, the prevalence of smoking (the number one preventable cause of death in the US) has declined from >50% in men and a >30% in women in the late 1960s, to about 25% in men and 20% in women, but it has not changed substantially in the last 5 years or so. In 2002 there were 48.5 million Americans who smoked (22.5% of the population).

In many ways, the prevalence of these risk factors is just a prelude to what is to follow, as these epidemic risk factors lead inexorably to even higher levels of CAD. Figure 1.11 further illustrates how these risk factors add incrementally to the risk of CHD in the Framingham study [19].

Growth Rate

From 1950 to 2000, the US population has grown from 152 million to 274 million, an annual rate of 1.2% per year and an increase of more than 120 million people. However, the growth was more rapid in the 1950s and 1960s—a reflection of the post WWII baby-boom (Table 1.2). Consequently, there has been a gradual increase in the percentage of the elderly as time passed. In 1950, 8.1% of the population were more than 65 years of age; by 2000 this had increased to 12.6% and is projected to increase even more dramatically by 2050 (Fig. 1.12). Despite the so-called baby-boom

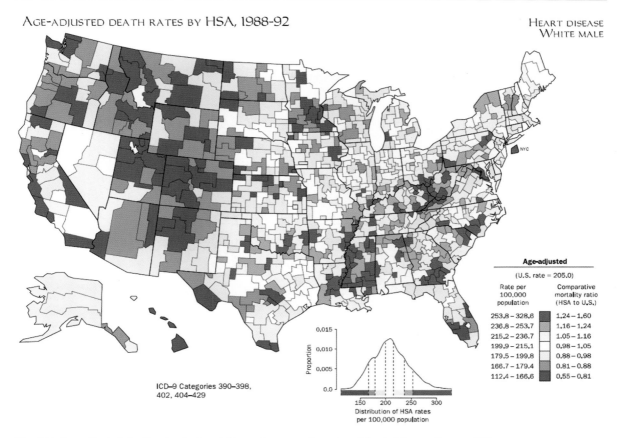

ICD–9 Categories 390–398,
402, 404–429

Fig. 1.5 Age-adjusted death rates for heart disease by age and gender. Adapted from reference [10]

"echo," as the baby-boomers in turn began having children in the 1980s and 1990s, the percentage of young children has declined. The first of the baby-boom generation, born in 1946, will be $\geq$65 years of age in 2011, and it is projected that the elderly proportion of the US population will continue to increase dramatically thereafter. In addition to the birth-rate impetus of the baby-boom, the life expectancy in the US has also risen in the last five decades, from 68.2 years in 1950 (59.1 in men, 62.9 in women) to 76.4 years in 2000 (64.6 in men, 74.7 in women). A lot of this has been attributable to the substantial decline in infant mortality in the 1950s and 1960s. Thus, the overall mortality rate alone may not provide a complete picture of the health demographics because it is strongly influenced by the age of the population; life expectancy is a more accurate reflection of the longevity of the population.

The death rate for heart disease has actually been declining over the past few decades, while the number of patients with CAD is increasing. This may reflect increasing quality of medical care, but it should be noted that in the elderly, heart disease becomes an ever more important cause of death, much more so than cancer. There are also concerns that while a lot of attention has been directed at smoking and cholesterol as risk factors, hypertension and diabetes are emerging as the next generation of major risk factors and are further accentuated in our increasingly obese and sedentary society.

A recent article by Foot et al. [20] attempted to project some of these trends into the near future and the more distant future. The near future projections (through 2010) are relatively easy because they are dominated by the existing population. The intermediate future (2010s and 2020s) is the period

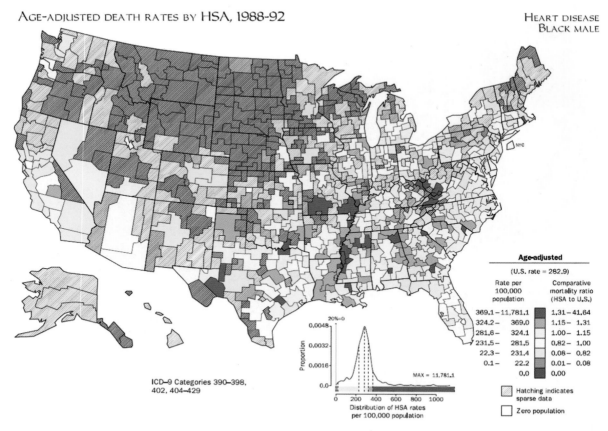

AGE-ADJUSTED DEATH RATES BY HSA, 1988-92

HEART DISEASE
BLACK MALE

ICD–9 Categories 390–398,
402, 404–429

Fig. 1.5 (continued)

in which the baby-boomers become the boomer-seniors. Finally, the longer-term future (2030s and 2040s) remains highly speculative and theoretical.

Any sort of projection requires assumptions, and population growth is a critical one. Foot et al. project three possible models: low (15% decrease in fertility across all ethnic groups), middle (fertility rates generally constant), and high (15% increase in fertility across all ethnic groups); similar assumptions in life expectancy and immigration rates are included. This gives rise to the US population projections in the year 2050 ranging from 282 million (low) to 394 million (middle) to 519 million (high). Interestingly, regardless of the projection used, all three models project that approximately 20% of the US population will be ≥65 years of age by the year 2050. This becomes particularly noteworthy when one considers that the rate of heart disease increases

exponentially with age increasing about tenfold between years 45–64 and 65+ (Table 1.3). Since the mid-1960s the rate of death has stabilized somewhat, and even started to decline recently, but the number of deaths, and more importantly the prevalence of disease, continues to increase.

Furthermore, with the development of revascularization strategies such as bypass surgery in the late 1960s and percutaneous revascularization in the late 1970s, more and more people with the disease are surviving longer and longer. Attempts to control risk factors such as hypertension, diabetes, smoking, and obesity have to some extent blunted exponential increases in life-threatening cardiac events, but do not reverse the disease process and do not eliminate the risk of adverse events, which continues to increase in our aging population.

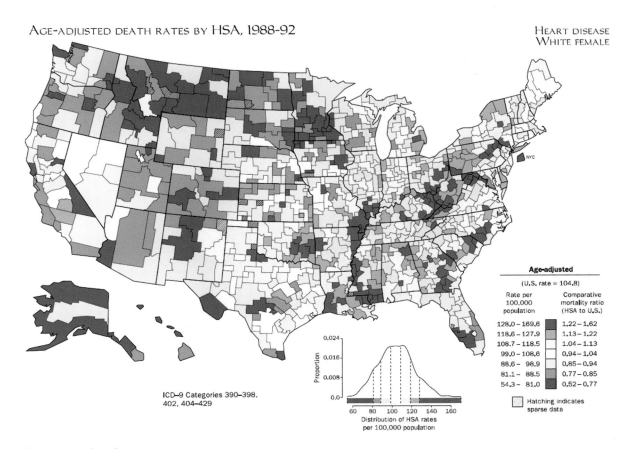

AGE-ADJUSTED DEATH RATES BY HSA, 1988-92

HEART DISEASE
WHITE FEMALE

ICD–9 Categories 390–398,
402, 404–429

Age-adjusted

(U.S. rate = 104.8)

Rate per 100,000 population	Comparative mortality ratio (HSA to U.S.)
128.0 – 169.6	1.22 – 1.62
118.6 – 127.9	1.13 – 1.22
108.7 – 118.5	1.04 – 1.13
99.0 – 108.6	0.94 – 1.04
88.6 – 98.9	0.85 – 0.94
81.1 – 88.5	0.77 – 0.85
54.3 – 81.0	0.52 – 0.77

Hatching indicates sparse data

Distribution of HSA rates per 100,000 population

Fig. 1.5 (continued)

The Burden

The increasing incidence of cardiac disease can therefore be attributed to both an increase in the population susceptible to the disease as well as an inability to curtail the risk factors for the disease. If anything, the risk factors for CAD are substantially *more* prevalent now. This increased incidence combines with the improved survival of afflicted individuals to result in an increasingly large number of patients with advanced disease.

The "burden" of chronic ischemic heart disease needs to be considered from a number of perspectives. First of all, there is the burden on the patient and the patient's family, who deal not only with the disease itself, but how it impacts on their lives and livelihoods. Next there is the burden to society as a whole, who must confront the costs associated with providing health care to an ever-growing population of patients. Finally, there is the burden to the health care system, not only from an economic standpoint, but also from a manpower standpoint; who is going to take care of all these people? How are they going to be trained? Not only will we need more physicians and more nurses, but we will also need more health professionals with cardiovascular expertise. Furthermore, with the ever-increasing technical complexity of care, we will need health professionals and health facilities with more complex techno-intense expertise. All of this comes at a cost—consider also that the therapeutic efforts at revascularization and risk factor reduction may reduce the likelihood of early cardiovascular events, but they increase the complexity of later events that may be superimposed on a pathophysiologically

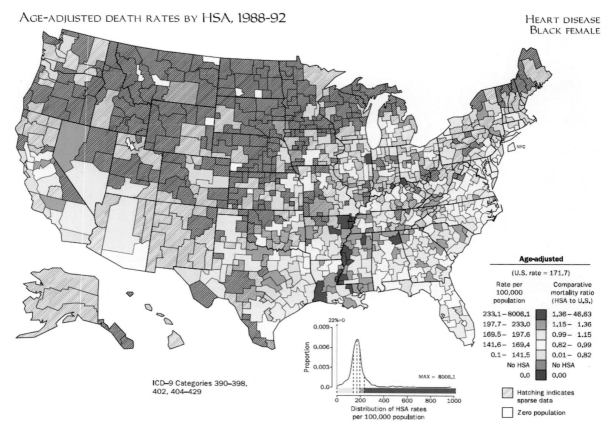

AGE-ADJUSTED DEATH RATES BY HSA, 1988-92

HEART DISEASE
BLACK FEMALE

ICD–9 Categories 390–398,
402, 404–429

Fig. 1.5 (continued)

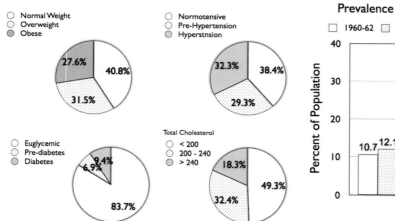

Fig. 1.6 Prevalence of risk factors for coronary artery disease. Adapted from reference [7]

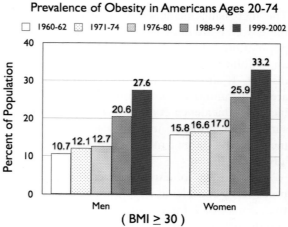

Fig. 1.7 Prevalence of obesity in the US by age groups. Adapted from references [11–15]

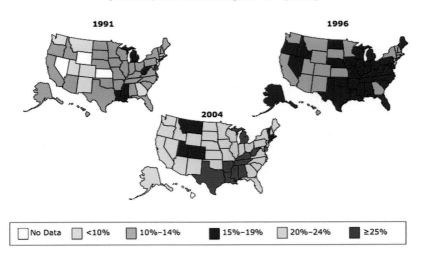

Fig. 1.8 Obesity trends in American adults. Adapted from references [11–15]

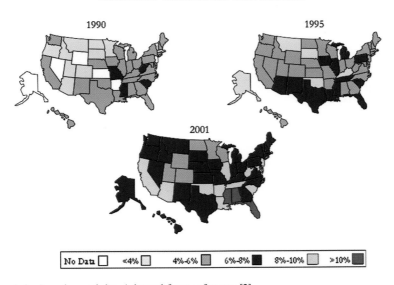

Fig. 1.9 Diabetes trends in American adults. Adapted from reference [2]

more complex foundation, namely more disease, later in life with more other ancillary medical problems complicating the procedure. In some ways we are victims of our own success, and success comes at a price; success also does not take the form of a *cure* for atherosclerosis, but rather in having our patients live longer with atherosclerotic disease. Even in the modern era, within 6 years of a first MI, 18% of men

and 35% of women will have a second MI, and 22% of men and 46% of women will be disabled by heart failure.

In 2005 it is estimated that the direct and indirect cost of coronary heart disease is US $142 billion. In 2002 there were an estimated 1,463,000 inpatient cardiac catheterizations, 515,000 CABG procedures, and 657,000 PCI

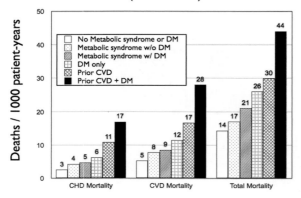

US Adult Mortality (NHANES II)

Fig. 1.10 Influence of diabetes and metabolic syndrome on cardiovascular mortality. Adapted from reference [19]

Table 1.1 Effects of additional risk factors in diabetics

8-year probability of CV events in diabetics (aged 50 years)		
Rate per 1,000	Women	Men
No other risk factors	50	54
HBP (≥165 mmHg)	117	139
HBP + Cholesterol > 260	159	213
HBP + Cholesterol + cigarettes	193	326
HBP + Cholesterol + cigarettes + ECG LVH	323	622

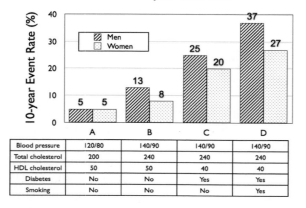

Estimated 10-year CHD Risk

	A	B	C	D
Blood pressure	120/80	140/90	140/90	140/90
Total cholesterol	200	240	240	240
HDL cholesterol	50	50	40	40
Diabetes	No	No	Yes	Yes
Smoking	No	No	No	Yes

Fig. 1.11 Influence of risk factors on cardiovascular mortality. Adapted from reference [20]

Table 1.2 The US population 1950–2000

	Number (in thousands)	Percent increase (%)
1950	152,271	14.5
1960	180,671	18.7
1970	250,052	13.5
1980	227,726	11.1
1990	249,949	9.8
2000	274,685	9.9

Adapted from reference [19].

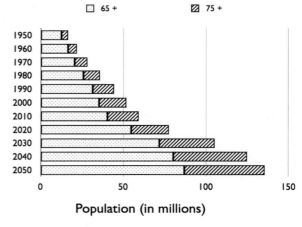

Projection US Elderly Population 1950-2050

Population (in millions)

Fig. 1.12 Projection of US elderly population. Adapted from reference [7]

Table 1.3 Heart disease deaths by age and gender in the US—1995

Age range (years)	Rank among causes of death	Total number of deaths Male	Female	Rate per 100,000 Male	Female
0–4	5	136	115	1.7	1.5
5–14	6	163	131	0.8	0.7
15–24	5	659	380	3.6	2.2
25–44	4	12,268	4,796	29.6	11.5
45–64	2	72,337	30,401	286.8	112.7
65+	1	276,756	338,670	2021.8	1706.7

Adapted from reference [19].

procedures. From 1979 to 2002 the number of cardiac catheterizations has increased almost fourfold; the number of PCI procedures has increased 324% since 1987. The total cost of cardiovascular disease and stroke is estimated to be almost $390 billion in 2005 [7]. Figure 1.13

Estimated Direct and Indirect Cost (in billions of dollars) Cardiovascular disease and Stroke United States 2005

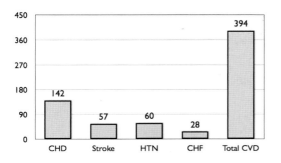

Fig. 1.13 Estimated direct and indirect costs (billions of dollars) of cardiovascular disease and stroke, US 2005

shows the breakdown of this cost for the individual components of coronary heart disease, stroke, hypertensive heart disease, and congestive heart failure. Outside the US, a recent study reported that the European Union spent 169 billion Euros in 2003 (equal to 181 billion Euros in 2005 prices) on cardiovascular disease. Of this, the approximately 2 million cardiovascular deaths that year accounted for 24.4 billion Euros, and the loss of 2.18 million working years. Put a different way, in 2003, this cost every man, woman, and child in the EU, 230 Euros, and involved significant restrictions of the daily activities of 4.4 million people, or one in every 100 people in the 25-nation EU. And these costs, are significantly below what the US spends, on the order of 715 Euros for every man, woman, and child [21].

If anything, the burdens that cardiovascular disease impose on our society are only going to get worse over the next few decades. Our population is getting older, has more risk factors, more disease, *and* more effective therapeutic options. We are caught between the Scylla of an emerging epidemic of ischemic heart disease as we get older, and the Charybdis of better therapies to reduce premature events and keep our patients alive longer.

Yes, Houston, we have a *real* problem. But, hopefully, fully grasping the scope of the problem is the first step in addressing it.

References

1. Lovell J and Kluger J. *Lost Moon: The Perilous Voyage of Apollo 13*. New York: Houghton Mifflin; 1994.
2. National Health and Nutrition Examination Survey (NHANES) http://www.cdc.gov/nchs/nhanes.html
3. Yang EH, Barsness GW, Gersh BJ, et al. Current and future treatment strategies for refractory angina. *Mayo Clin Proc* 2004; 79(10): 1284–92.
4. Strong K, Mathers C, Leeder S, Beaglehole R. Preventing chronic diseases: how many lives can we save? *Lancet* 2005; 366: 1578.
5. Cupples LA, D'Agostino RB, Kiely D. The Framingham Heart Study, Section 35: An Epidemiological Investigation of Cardiovascular Disease: Survival Following Cardiovascular Events: 30-Year Follow-up. Bethesda, MD: National Heart Lung and Blood Institute; 1988.
6. Anderson RN, Smith BL. Deaths: leading causes for 2002. *NVSR* 2005; 53(17): 90. (PHS) 2005–1120.
7. American Heart Association. *Heart disease and stroke statistics – 2005 update*. Dallas, TX: American Heart Association.
8. American Heart Association. *Heart disease and stroke statistics – 2008 update*. Dallas, TX: American Heart Association.
9. Sharrett AR, Ballantyne CM, Coady SA, et al. Coronary heart disease prediction from lipoprotein cholesterol levels, triglycerides, lipoprotein (a), apolipoproteins A-I and B, and HDL density subfractions: the Atherosclerosis Risk in Communities (ARIC) study. *Circulation* 2001; 104: 1108–13.
10. CDC/NCHS Atlas of United States Mortality. http://www.cdc.gov/nchs/data/gis/atmaphd.pdf
11. Mokdad AH, Serdula MK, Dietz WH, et al. The spread of the obesity epidemic in the United States, 1991–1998. *JAMA* 1999; 282: 1519–22.
12. Mokdad AH, Ford ES, Bowman BA, et al. Diabetes trends in the US: 1990–1998. *Diabetes Care* 2000; 23: 1278–83.
13. Mokdad AH, Bowman BA, Ford ES, et al. The continuing epidemic of obesity and diabetes in the United States. *JAMA* 2001; 286: 1195–200.
14. Mokdad AH, Ford ES, Bowman BA, et al. Prevalence of obesity, diabetes, and obesity-related health risk factors, 2001. *JAMA* 2003; 289: 76–9.
15. CDC Behavioral Risk Factor Surveillance System (BRFSS); http://aps.ncdd.cdc.gov/brfss
16. The STOPP-T2D Prevention Study Group. Presence of diabetes risk factors in a large US eighth-grade cohort. *Diabetes Care* 2006; 29: 121–217.
17. Malik S, Wong ND, Franklin SS, et al. Impact of the metabolic syndrome on mortality from coronary heart disease, cardiovascular disease, and all causes in United States adults. *Circulation* 2004; 110: 1245–50.
18. National Cholesterol Education Program (NCEP) Expert Panel on Detection, Evaluation, and Treatment of High Blood Cholesterol in Adults (Adult Treatment Panel III). Third Report of the National Cholesterol

Education Program (NCEP) Expert Panel on Detection, Evaluation, and Treatment of High Blood Cholesterol in Adults (Adult Treatment Panel III) final report. *Circulation* 2002; 106: 3143–421.

19. Wilson PW, D'Agostino RB, Levy D, et al. Prediction of coronary heart disease using risk factor categories. *Circulation* 1998; 97(18): 1837–47.

20. Foot DK, Lewis RP, Pearson TA, Beller GB. Demographics and cardiology, 1950–2050. *J Am Coll Cardiol* 2000; 35: 1067–81.

21. Leal J, Luengo-Fernandez R, Gray A. Economic burden of cardiovascular diseases in the enlarged European Union. *Eur Heart J* 2006; 27: 1610–9. (http//eurheartj. oxfordjournals.org)

Chapter 2
Imaging for Viable and Ischemic Myocardium

Value of Assessment of Viable and Ischemic Myocardium and Techniques Such as MRI, Radionuclide Imaging

Catalin Loghin and K. Lance Gould

Introduction

Myocardial ischemia and infarction cause abnorma myocardial metabolism, decreased left ventricular (LV) systolic function, diastolic dysfunction, congestive heart failure, and decreased survival. Consequently, revascularization techniques, either surgical or catheter based, have become integral to treatment of severe ischemic heart disease.

With revascularization, significant areas of dysfunctional myocardium can regain their function, resulting in improved LV performance and in increased survival. Current data suggests that 25–40% of patients with ischemic LV dysfunction are potential candidates for improvement following revascularization [1–5]. The challenge lies in correctly identifying this group of patients based on accurate detection of ischemic and viable myocardium.

Nuclear imaging techniques, like single photon emission tomography (SPECT) and positron emission tomography (PET), directly assess myocardial perfusion, cell membrane integrity, cellular metabolism, and the molecular mechanisms of ischemic viable or necrotic myocardium, thereby indicating revascularization procedures or not.

Historical Perspective and Definitions

Over the past 25 years, the basis for revascularization of dysfunctional injured myocardium has undergone major changes. In the initial years of quantifying LV function, its impairment at resting conditions was regarded as an irreversible process of myocardial necrosis and scarring. However, early observations from Heyndrickx GR et al. showed experimentally that regional myocardial dysfunction could persist for hours after coronary occlusion followed by recovery of function with reperfusion in the absence of myocardial infarction (MI) [6]. This delayed recovery of contractility was later called "stunned myocardium" [7]. The concept of stunned myocardium was then extended to repetitive short episodes of severe myocardial ischemia, followed by adequate myocardial perfusion after the transient ischemic period.

The concept of "hibernating myocardium" was later reported based on clinical observations rather than animal experiments [8, 9] as persistent, stable hypoperfusion, and ischemia leading to a chronic state of poor LV contractility that was reversible with revascularization or restoration of adequate coronary flow. Hibernating and stunned myocardium are both characterized by poorly contracting myocardium that is viable (alive) myocardium that recovers contractile function after revascularization, in contrast to permanently dysfunctional scar tissue. Finally, the concept of "ischemic preconditioning" was first described experimentally in dogs when short repetitive episodes of myocardial ischemia resulted in reduced infarction following a subsequent prolonged coronary artery occlusion [10].

Stunning, hibernation and ischemic preconditioning are all elements of acute or chronic heart

C. Loghin (✉)
Division of Cardiology, University of Texas Health Science
Center, Houston, TX, USA
e-mail: catalin.loghin@uth.tmc.edu

R. Delgado, H.S. Arora (eds.), *Interventional Treatment of Advanced Ischemic Heart Disease*,
DOI 10.1007/978-1-84800-395-8_2, © Springer-Verlag London Limited 2009

adaptation to severe temporary or persistent ischemia that contribute to the preservation of the myocyte structural and functional integrity [11] by reducing regional myocardial oxygen consumption in the face of limited blood supply. Ischemic tissue is viable with preserved contractility under resting conditions as opposed to stunned and hibernating myocardium that is viable with impaired contraction.

The term "myocardial viability" is defined functionally as the capacity of ischemically injured, non-contracting myocardium to recover contractile function after revascularization or reperfusion [12]. The term refers to both acute dysfunction (stunned myocardium) and a chronic state low resting perfusion (hibernating myocardium), both of which indicate revascularization and consequent improved cardiac contraction. This functional definition is based on the outcome of revascularization in retrospect and does not refer to specific biological processes or cell behavior that predicts recovery of LV function. Identifying any of several different cellular processes of viable or "live" but non-contractile myocardium by imaging or functional testing then becomes the basis for revascularization procedures expected to improve contractile function. Therefore, the term is defined by the specific imaging technology used to determine "viability", such as by nuclear methods to image cell membrane integrity and metabolism or alternatively by low dose dobutamine echocardiography or magnetic resonance imaging of reserve contractility. Nuclear cardiology has evolved in parallel with our understanding of the myocardial response to severe ischemia from imaging markers of the myocyte potassium space by late redistribution imaging [13] to metabolic imaging for separating viable from necrotic or scarred myocardium to the concept of reverse redistribution as a marker of endothelial dysfunction in advanced or early coronary artery disease before significant ischemia develops [14] and finally to molecular imaging.

Physiologic Principles of Myocardial Perfusion Imaging

The well established phenomenon of "perfusion-contraction matching" [15] is an adaptive myocardial response to chronically diminished perfusion. Therefore, analyzing this adaptive process requires simultaneous study of myocardial perfusion, metabolism, and regional myocardial function. The physiologic principles of myocardial perfusion imaging (MPI) with SPECT and PET imaging for identifying or assessing severity of coronary artery stenosis and ischemia derive from the concepts of coronary flow reserve [16–23].

Flow through moderately severe coronary artery stenosis is commonly normal at rest but becomes inadequate for the increased metabolic requirements and blood flow during stress. Coronary blood flow normally increases to four times resting baseline flow rates after coronary artery vasodilators such as dipyridamole and adenosine. A stenosis restricts maximal blood flow capacity compared to normal coronary arteries, thereby causing a disparity in regional perfusion of areas supplied by a stenotic artery compared to normal coronary arteries. This disparity manifests as a relative perfusion defect during stress, corresponding to the ischemic myocardial territory supplied by a stenotic artery. Furthermore, the quantitative severity of the relative perfusion defect is proportional to the severity of the stenosis under conditions of maximal coronary flow after dipyridamole or adenosine stress [24].

Figure 2.1 illustrates normal myocardial perfusion by PET using ^{82}Rubidium (^{82}Rb) at rest and after dipyridamole stress in 3D views. A coronary arterial map is overlaid on the perfusion image or alternatively an arterial distribution map as a precise perfusion atlas of the coronary artery tree and all its secondary and tertiary branches [25].

In Fig. 2.2, the PET perfusion images show severe stenosis or occlusion of the left circumflex (LCx) and right (RCA) coronary arteries with a moderately severe stenosis of the left anterior descending (LAD) coronary artery proximal to its second diagonal branch. The ejection fraction (EF) and regional LV contraction were normal. Therefore, this example illustrates purely ischemic myocardium without scar and without injured or poorly contracting myocardium.

With single photon emission computed tomography (SPECT), an average difference from normal to abnormal regions of 30–50% is necessary before the abnormality is visually identifiable [17], as opposed to PET where differences of only 5–10% can be visually detected. Moreover, PET has the unique ability to non-invasively quantify relative or absolute coronary blood flow and metabolism

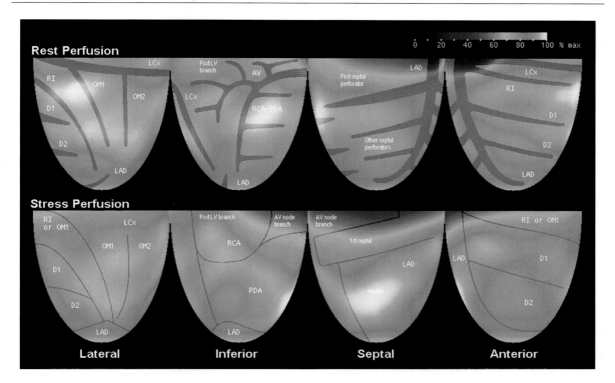

Fig. 2.1 Normal myocardial perfusion by positron emission tomography using ^{82}Rubidium (^{82}Rb) at rest and after dipyridamole stress in 3D views. Coronary arterial maps are superimposed. Perfusion is displayed on a color scale, representing fraction of normal perfusion

based on quantitative measurements of myocardial radionuclide uptake without attenuation artifacts that limit SPECT.

In contrast to imaging relative coronary reserve during stress for ischemia due to flow limiting stenosis, assessing viability requires imaging metabolic processes and perfusion at resting conditions. Both SPECT and PET can be used to evaluate direct measures of myocardial viability by imaging intermediary metabolism and/or the potassium space reflecting cell membrane function. However, PET is more accurate due to higher resolution and correction of attenuation defects. By comparison, dobutamine stress echocardiography and magnetic resonance imaging (MRI) evaluate the reserve contractile capacity of the heart during stress as an indirect measure of myocardial viability.

Non-contracting viable myocardium traps potassium analogues in the myocyte potassium space, such as ^{201}Thallium (^{201}Tl) for SPECT imaging and ^{82}Rb for PET imaging, reflecting sufficient cell membrane integrity [4, 26–32] to maintain the intracellular potassium space. Therefore, residual trapping of these potassium analogue radiotracers identifies viable myocardium associated with recovery of contraction following revascularization.

For SPECT, ^{201}Tl is the most useful tracer for viability assessment, since it is a potassium analog pooling in the intracellular potassium space. After initial cellular uptake of ^{201}Tl in approximate proportion to perfusion, a continuous exchange of the tracer occurs between the blood pool, the extracellular space, and the intracellular space. This exchange is the basis for ^{201}Tl redistribution to underperfused regions with delayed trapping in the potassium space. In viable myocardium with persistent low coronary flow, ^{201}Tl slowly redistributes into the resting perfusion defect, thereby making it less severe or even normalizing on late 4–24 h resting images.

Redistribution imaging may be combined with stress. If a resting defect persists with late

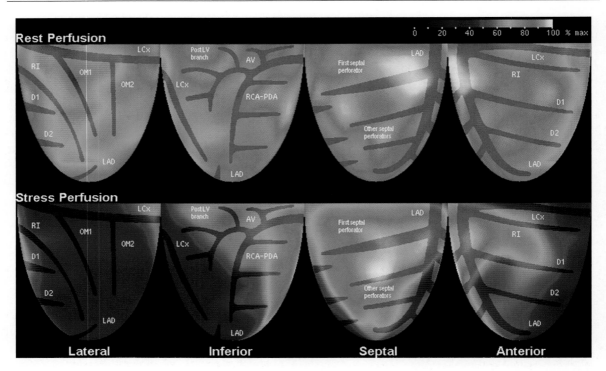

Fig. 2.2 Positron emission tomography (PET) perfusion images showing severe stenosis/ occlusion of the left circumflex (LCx) and right (RCA) coronary arteries with a moderately severe stenosis of the left anterior descending (LAD) coronary artery

redistribution imaging, a second dose of ^{201}Tl may be injected with repeat imaging 6–24 h later. With this re-injection technique, up to 49% of the fixed defects on late redistribution imaging will show normal or improved uptake, suggesting viability [33].

While ^{201}Tl is optimal for SPECT imaging of viable myocardium, Technetium-99m-sestamibi (MIBI) may also be used. MIBI distribution reflects regional blood flow and requires preserved cellular membrane and mitochondrial function for uptake and intracellular retention [34–36]. However, as compared to ^{201}Tl, MIBI does not demonstrate redistribution and viability is based on initial uptake rather than on defect reversibility with delayed imaging. Since MIBI is more easily produced than ^{201}Tl, it is more commonly used for stress perfusion imaging as well as viability. The use of ECG gated perfusion images of MIBI or ^{201}Tl to assess LV wall motion (gated SPECT) may increase the accuracy of viability assessment [37]. The addition of nitrates to enhance restng perfusion may also increase diagnostic sensitivity [38].

Dual isotope SPECT protocols obtain resting images with ^{201}Tl and stress images with MIBI followed by 24 h ^{201}Tl late redistribution imaging [39, 40]. These protocols have demonstrated good prediction of contractile function recovery after revascularization comparable to simpler single tracer protocols [41].

While SPECT imaging with ^{201}Tl and MIBI is commonly used to demonstrate viability, these technologies may provide incorrect information in approximately 20% of patients with large severe defects and low EF. PET is the gold standard for assessing viability due to its higher resolution, attenuation correction, and quantification of radionuclide uptake. Moreover, PET can demonstrate cell membrane integrity with the potassium analog ^{82}Rb and uptake of metabolic tracers using radiolabeled glucose, fatty acids, and acetate or oxygen analogs.

With adequate blood flow and oxygen supply after fasting or a fatty meal, normal myocardium metabolizes primarily fatty acids while glucose metabolism is suppressed. Therefore, normally contracting, normally perfused myocardium does not take up glucose or its radio-labeled analogues like ^{18}F-fluoro-2-deoxyglucose (FDG) under fasting conditions or after a fatty meal. Failure of myocardial FDG uptake due to preferential fatty acids metabolism may cause defects on an FDG image that look the same as a myocardial scar. Consequently, imaging with FDG is done after a high carbohydrate meal and oral glucose load that shifts normal myocardium from fatty acids to glucose metabolism such that normal and ischemic viable myocardium take up FDG but necrotic or scarred myocardium does not, appearing as a defect.

In ischemic viable myocytes, the lack of oxygen inhibits fatty acids oxidation and myocardial metabolism is shifted toward anaerobic glycolysis of glucose. Therefore, under fed conditions after a high carbohydrate meal or after an oral glucose load, areas of hibernating myocardium with low perfusion will preferentially take up FDG resulting in a metabolism–perfusion mismatch (high FDG uptake, low perfusion) as a marker of viable hypoperfused dysfunctional myocardium [42–44]. Surrounding normal myocardium will also take up FDG but will have normal perfusion and function. Regions of stunned myocardium also demonstrate normal or enhanced glucose uptake but the resting perfusion is normal in areas of poorly contracting myocardium [45]. However, with stunned myocardium, stress perfusion images have a severe stress induced perfusion defect as the cause of repetitive ischemia leading to contractile dysfunction.

Residual trapping of metabolic analogues by hibernating myocardium, such as FDG [46–48], ^{11}Carbon (^{11}C) acetate [49–52], and ^{11}C palmitate [53–55] reflects sufficient integrity of myocytes and their metabolism to allow recovery of myocardial contractile function after revascularization.

Of these metabolic analogues, FDG has been the most extensively studied and is the most widely used PET marker of myocardial viability [56]. FDG is transported across the myocyte cell membrane and is phosphorylated by hexokinase. The phosphorylated compound cannot be metabolized or transported out of the cell and is therefore trapped in the myocyte. However, under some conditions,

FDG studies may not accurately predict contractility recovery, since FDG uptake also depends on fasting or fed state, insulin and serum fatty acids levels, insulin resistance, cardiac work, catecholamines, and pH [57–60]. Good FDG PET images of the heart can be routinely obtained by having patients eat a carbohydrate meal, giving a glucose load, with insulin in diabetics, and avoiding catecholamine stimulus such as aminophylline after pharmacologic stress.

Concomitant with PET imaging of FDG, myocardial perfusion is imaged with ^{13}N-ammonia [61–63] or with ^{82}Rb [64]. The combined perfusion FDG images demonstrate several patterns:

(i) matched normal flow and metabolism in normal myocardium with normal perfusion and normal function;
(ii) matched normal flow and metabolism in normal myocardium with reduced regional contractile function characteristic of stunned myocardium or, if global, typical of cardiomyopathy;
(iii) matched defects on both perfusion and metabolic images showing diminished flow and diminished metabolism consistent with scar tissue;
(iv) the perfusion-metabolism mismatch pattern, with reduced coronary flow and normal/increased FDG uptake, characteristic of viable hibernating myocardium;
(v) reversed perfusion metabolism mismatch with normal perfusion, reduced FDG uptake and normal function that is due to preferential fatty acids metabolism in non-ischemic myocardium. However, if contractile function is reduced, this reverse mismatch may also indicate stunned myocardium with normal fatty acids metabolism that recovers quickly after restored perfusion, whereas recovery of contractile function may require weeks to months [65].

Figure 2.3 illustrates PET images of resting perfusion and metabolism using FDG showing a large myocardial scar in the LAD proximal to the first septal perforator that wraps around the apex and up the infero-apical wall. The scar is characterized by low perfusion and low metabolism or low FDG uptake (perfusion–metabolism match with low uptake of both radionuclides). The distribution of the LCx is mildly hypoperfused at rest but active metabolically with FDG uptake, thereby indicating

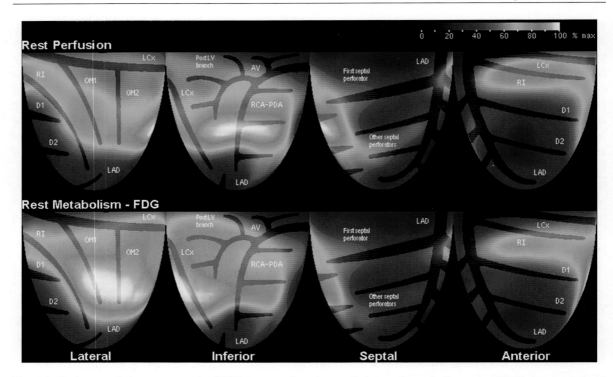

Fig. 2.3 Positron emission tomography (PET) images of resting perfusion and metabolism using FDG showing a large myocardial scar in the LAD proximal to the first septal perforator

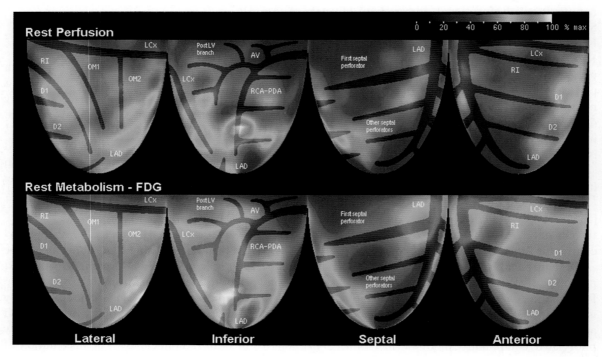

Fig. 2.4 PET images showing hibernating myocardium with low resting perfusion but active metabolism with normal FDG uptake in the distribution of the LCx and the diagonal branches off the LAD (perfusion-metabolism mismatch). There is also a septal scar

that it is viable. The ramus intermedius (RI) and the RCA are normally perfused at resting conditions with normal metabolic uptake of FDG (perfusion–metabolism match—normal perfusion and metabolism).

Figure 2.4 illustrates hibernating myocardium with low resting perfusion but active metabolism with normal FDG uptake in the distribution of the LCx and the diagonal branches of the LAD (perfusion–metabolism mismatch). There is scar with low perfusion and low FDG uptake in septum (perfusion–metabolism match—low perfusion and low metabolism) indicating scar.

Figure 2.5 illustrates still another combination of metabolic states of clinical importance. There is hibernating myocardium (mismatch with low perfusion and normal metabolic FDG uptake) in the distribution of the mid LAD wrapping around the apex with scar (matched low perfusion and low metabolism—low FDG uptake) in the RCA distribution. In the distribution of the LCx and proximal LAD including the first septal perforator, the

perfusion is high and FDG uptake is low due to such good blood perfusion that the myocardium burns free fatty acids rather than taking up the glucose analog FDG.

Figure 2.6 illustrates stunned myocardium with normal resting perfusion but a severe stress induced perfusion defect that indicates severe ischemia in the distribution of the RCA and the LAD proximal to the first septal perforator. Metabolic imaging with FDG is not necessary, since resting perfusion is normal without scar with a left ventricular ejection fraction (LVEF) of 30% thereby indicating stunned myocardium that normalized after bypass surgery. This patient with severe stress induced ischemia and reduced LV function characteristic of stunned myocardium contrasts with the patient of Fig. 2.2 with severe ischemia but normal LV function and no stunning.

Figure 2.7 also illustrates stunned myocardium with resting perfusion and resting metabolic uptake of FDG in a patient with congestive heart failure, diabetes, and a LVEF of 10% where stress was not

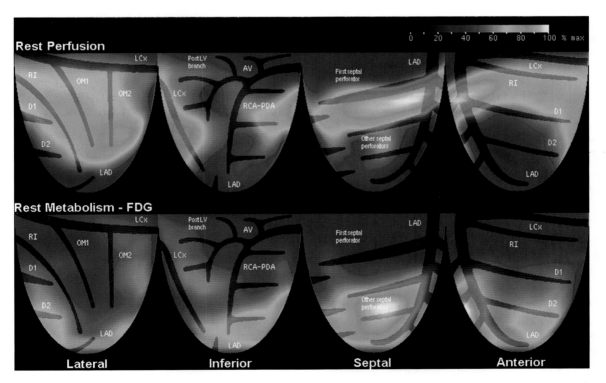

Fig. 2.5 Positron emission tomography (PET) scan showing hibernating myocardium (mismatch with low perfusion and normal metabolic FDG uptake) in the distribution of the mid LAD with scar (matched low perfusion and low metabolism—low FDG uptake) in the RCA distribution

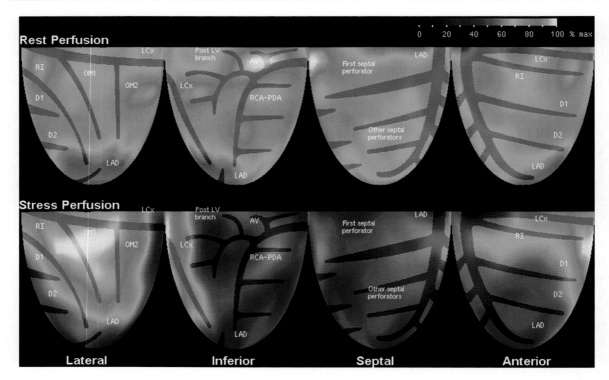

Fig. 2.6 Positron emission tomography (PET) scan showing stunned myocardium with normal resting perfusion but a severe stress induced perfusion defect that indicates severe ischemia in the distribution of the RCA and the LAD proximal to the first septal perforator. See text for details

done due to known severe three-vessel disease by prior coronary arteriography. Resting perfusion is mildly reduced in the distribution of the LCx and second diagonal branch of the LAD with normal resting perfusion throughout the rest of the LV. Such mild hypoperfusion of a relatively modestly sized area would not reduce the LVEF to 10% leaving the conclusion that the low LVEF was due to stunning associated with severe three-vessel disease. After 6 vessel bypass surgery the CHF resolved and LVEF improved to 40%, suggesting an element of cardiomyopathy that accounted for the remaining mildly impaired contractility.

Despite addressing different cellular functions, imaging the potassium space by [82]Rb or by cellular metabolic trapping of FDG, the size and severity of the defects obtained with both radionuclides by PET are virtually identical [66, 67], indicating equivalent preservation of these two measures of viability.

Radionuclide Imaging of Chronic Ischemic Heart Disease

For patients with chronic CAD, nuclear imaging is essential for addressing the following major clinical issues: (i) detection of ischemic myocardium, (ii) differentiation between viable hibernating or stunned myocardium and scar tissue in mechanically dysfunctional regions, and (iii) risk stratification for future major adverse events. Such information provides the basis for percutaneous coronary intervention (PCI) or coronary artery bypass (CAB) surgery and assessing their outcomes based on detection of residual ischemia and recovery of contractile function.

Indications for radionuclide imaging in these patients are detailed in current ACC/AHA guidelines [68] and ACCF/ASNC appropriateness criteria for SPECT myocardial perfusion imaging [69]. While a detailed discussion of these indications is beyond the purpose of this text, for patients with advanced

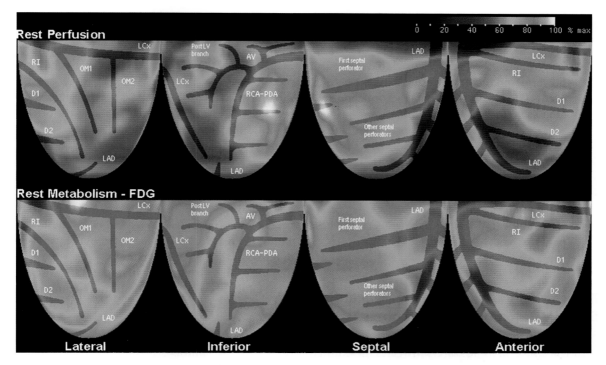

Fig. 2.7 Positron emission tomography (PET) scan showing resting perfusion and resting metabolic uptake of FDG in a patient with congestive heart failure. There is mildly reduced resting perfusion in the distribution of the LCx and second diagonal branch of the LAD

ischemic heart disease and LV dysfunction, these guidelines emphasize the following:

(i) Detection of ischemic myocardium: for symptomatic patients at risk for or with known CAD an MPI study is warranted, either by SPECT of by PET, if the patient can tolerate a form of stress and if cardiac catheterization is not the most appropriate initial test as for acute unstable coronary syndromes. For asymptomatic patients, radionuclide imaging with stress to detect ischemia is appropriate for the following categories: (a) new onset or known heart failure or LV systolic dysfunction if there is no prior CAD evaluation and no cardiac catheterization is planned for other reasons and (b) in patients at greater than or equal to 5 years after CAB and at 2 years after PCI [69].

(ii) Viability assessment: SPECT or PET imaging are indicated in patients with known CAD after myocardial infarction or by cardiac catheterization with dysfunctional myocardial segments by echocardiography, radionuclide angiography or gated SPECT. Any viability imaging protocol should address the presence of coexistent ischemia as well as of regional wall motion abnormalities and LV global systolic performance.

(iii) Evaluation of risk for future events: the combined assessment of myocardial ischemia and of the amount of scar and viable tissue represents a powerful tool in predicting outcomes of patients with ischemic heart disease.

Size and severity of ischemic areas correlate well with mortality in both stable CAD populations [70] and after myocardial infarction [71]. Moreover, the presence of ischemia in a dysfunctional segment of myocardium is a powerful predictor of functional recovery. Up to 83% of regions with reversible defects (ischemia) will improve with revascularization compared to only 33% for regions where no reversibility was demonstrated [72]. In patients with heart failure, viable poorly contracting myocardium correlates with recovery of regional [73] and global LV function [74] after revascularization with improvement of functional heart failure class [75]. For post MI patients, the presence of viable tissue is a powerful predictor of future adverse cardiac events [76, 77] that warrants radionuclide imaging as a guide to revascularization.

(iv) After revascularization, appropriate indications for MPI include patients who present with a chest pain syndrome, or are asymptomatic but at greater than 5 years after CAB or 2 years after PCI [69]. Radionuclide ventriculography or gated perfusion imaging is useful to evaluate LV functional recovery in these patients.

Myocardial Viability, Size of Myocardial Scar, LV Function, and Outcomes

Positron emission tomography provides the optimal basis for clinical decisions on revascularization of patients with impaired LV function and for reducing the number of unnecessary procedures. Overall, PET positive and negative accuracy for predicting improved LV function is 85–90% [78].

In post myocardial infarction patients, LVEF is closely related to the infarct size by PET, as illustrated in Fig. 2.8 [79]. In such patients, the presence of viable myocardium is associated with good survival post revascularization, whereas the absence of viable

myocardium predicts a higher mortality rate that is not improved by revascularization. Thus, appropriate evaluation for presence of viable myocardium can exclude patients from unnecessary revascularization procedures.

Almost half (46%) of all post MI patients will have completed necrosis without remaining areas of viable myocardium; of the remaining 54%, some will benefit from revascularization or from vigorous reversal treatment of atherosclerosis [79, 80], summarized by Fig. 2.9. The benefit of revascularization has been well established only in patients with moderate LV dysfunction (LVEF < 35%), whereas the survival benefit for those with regional LV dysfunction without reduced LVEF is suggested only by non-randomized or uncontrolled studies [81].

The challenge consists of identifying those at high enough risk, with a substantial amount of viable myocardium, who would benefit from revascularization. The criteria for selecting such patients include symptoms, collaterals, LV function, ischemic burden, associated indications for cardiovascular surgery or co-morbidities, and the amount of viable myocardium.

Much of the research on myocardial viability has focused on measuring pathological changes, cellular metabolism, or myocardial contractility without defining how much of the myocardium is involved, its relation to LV systolic function, and clinical outcomes. PET currently provides the best answer to the following questions: (a) How much myocardium is scarred or viable as a percent of the zone at risk distal to a stenosis and as a percent of the whole heart? (b) What amount of viable tissue justifies revascularization?

The zone at risk is defined differently from the infarct area and from viability as the area of reduced flow reserve by dipyridamole stress perfusion imaging rather than by rest perfusion imaging. The physiologic basis for this approach is the well documented observation that resting coronary flow may be normal with up to 85% stenosis; consequently, rest imaging may not define the correct size of zone at risk, as illustrated by the example below.

There is a conceptual difference between myocardial viability in a resting perfusion defect versus a stress induced defect. A rest perfusion defect may enlarge peripherally with stress due to reduced flow reserve secondary to a flow limiting stenosis,

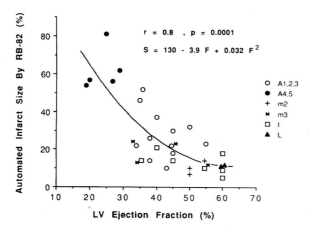

Fig. 2.8 Relationship between left ventricular ejection fraction and infarct size by PET

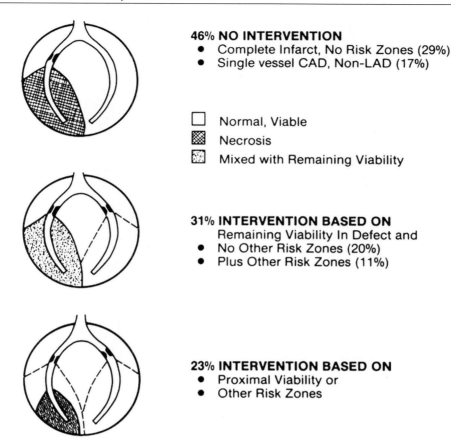

46% **NO INTERVENTION**
- Complete Infarct, No Risk Zones (29%)
- Single vessel CAD, Non-LAD (17%)

☐ Normal, Viable
▨ Necrosis
▨ Mixed with Remaining Viability

31% **INTERVENTION BASED ON**
Remaining Viability In Defect and
- No Other Risk Zones (20%)
- Plus Other Risk Zones (11%)

23% **INTERVENTION BASED ON**
- Proximal Viability or
- Other Risk Zones

Fig. 2.9 Effect of revascularization on myocardial viability in post myocardial infarction (MI) patients. Almost half of all post MI patients will have completed necrosis without remaining areas of viable myocardium

defining a border zone at risk that is by definition viable myocardium. However, in this situation there is no information on viability of the central area of the resting defect that may be either scar or partial scar mixed with viable (hibernating or stunned) myocardium. Incorrect definition of the size of the zone at risk, scar, and amount of viable myocardium leads to unnecessary revascularization in 31–39% of the patients undergoing such procedures [77, 79, 82, 83].

Figure 2.10 illustrates a zone at risk by PET perfusion imaging. In this example, there is a moderate resting perfusion defect indicating a small non-transmural scar in the distribution of the LAD. After dipyridamole stress, the perfusion defect becomes larger and more severe, indicating a large border zone of ischemic myocardium around the small scar supplied by a severe stenosis. The border zone area is large enough to justify revascularization without metabolic imaging in this instance.

The different stages of ischemic dysfunctional myocardium are a continuum of regional rest or stress-induced hypoperfusion, cell membrane integrity (^{201}Tl and ^{82}Rb uptake), metabolic changes (FDG uptake), preserved, absent, or inducible contractility (dobutamine echocardiography or MRI), variable degrees of myocyte dedifferentiation [84], and tissue fibrosis. The degree to which each of these elements is impaired defines the specific conditions of ischemic, stunned, and hibernating myocardium (all viable tissue states) and scar (non-viable tissue) for a particular myocardial region. Moreover, for a particular region of the myocardium, two or more of these conditions usually coexist, such as scar mixed with ischemia

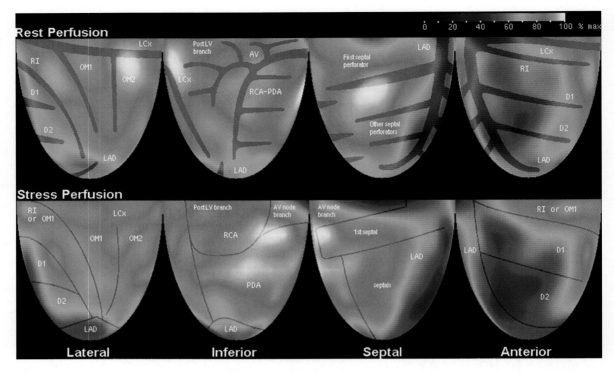

Fig. 2.10 Positron emission tomography (PET) perfusion images showing a "zone at risk." There is a moderate resting perfusion defect indicating a small non-transmural scar in the distribution of the LAD. After dipyridamole stress, the perfusion defect becomes larger and more severe, indicating a large border zone of ischemic myocardium around the small scar supplied by a severe stenosis

or ischemic tissue mixed with non-contractile but viable myocardium or a mix of all three.

Therefore, various methods used for viability testing may provide somewhat discordant predictions of the recovery of contractile function after revascularization, as demonstrated by Bax JJ et al. [85, 86]. In an early comparative study, FDG PET and ^{201}Tl had the highest weighted mean sensitivity (88% and 90%, respectively) in predicting myocardial functional recovery, whereas FDG PET and low dose dobutamine echocardiography had the highest specificity (73% and 81%, respectively) [86]. The overall accuracy of different viability methods in predicting recovery with revascularization ranges between 66% and 81% [87].

However, another large meta-analysis study found no difference between different viability testing methods for predicting survival after revascularization, suggesting that decisions driven by viability studies are clinically equivalent and have similar outcomes, irrespective of the technique used [88]. While improved LV function is a major factor affecting

survival, reduced risk of arrhythmia and reduced rate of acute coronary syndromes and/or heart failure symptoms may contribute to the overall benefit.

While this chapter focuses on myocardium that will benefit from revascularization procedure, vigorous treatment of risk factors is essential for stopping progression of the atherosclerosis in native or coronary bypasses. The patient in Fig. 2.11 is a physician who had a myocardial infarction leading to coronary bypass surgery. The PET scan in Fig. 2.11 was obtained a year after bypass surgery, showing a severe resting (top row) defect of the apex in the distribution of the initial LAD occlusion. Dipyridamole stress causes more severe larger perfusion defects (middle row) in the distribution of the LAD and a large LCX, indicating severe residual diffuse coronary artery disease. The lower row of Fig. 2.11 shows the rest and dipyridamole stress perfusion images after 10 years of vigorous lifestyle and pharmacologic management including food with 10% of calories as fat, maintenance of lean

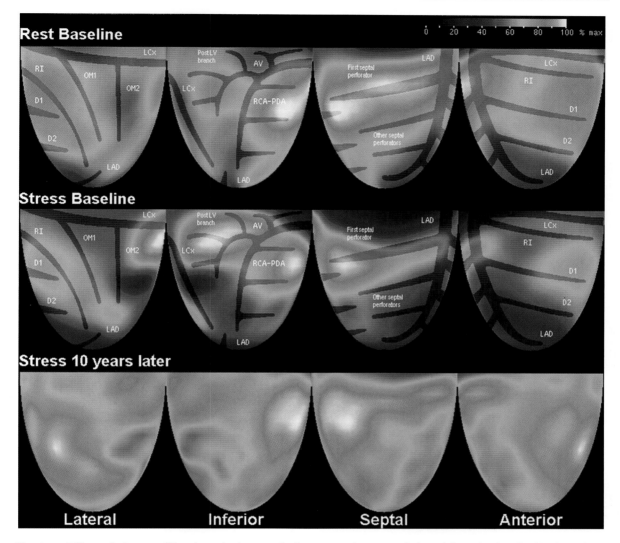

Fig. 2.11 Effect of vigorous lifestyle and pharmacologic management on stopping progression of CAD. *Top row*: PET scan a year after bypass surgery, showing a severe resting defect of the apex in the distribution of the initial LAD occlusion. *Middle row*: Dipyridamole stress causes more severe larger perfusion defects in the distribution of the LAD and a large LCx, indicating severe residual diffuse coronary artery disease. *Lower row*: Dipyridamole stress perfusion images after 10 years showing marked improvement of the diffuse disease

body weight, daily workouts, Zocor 20 mg and Niaspan 1,500 mg daily to maintain total cholesterol 136 mg/dl, triglycerides 65 mg/dl, LDL 58 mg/dl, and HDL 65 mg/dl. Interim PET scans showed steady improvement up to this 10-year follow-up scan with progressively marked improvement of the diffuse disease that initially caused severe defects despite open bypass grafts.

Not all severe perfusion defects require revascularization procedures for patients with stable, even severe, angina who prefer vigorous medical treatment. In Fig. 2.12, the rest perfusion image (upper row) shows a small transmural scar in the distribution of the distal LCx that is more severe and larger after dipyridamole stress (middle row). Quantitative analysis showed myocardial steal in the region of the defect, indicating collateralization to the LCX beyond an occlusion, confirmed by coronary arteriography. After reviewing the options and risks, the patient undertook a strict

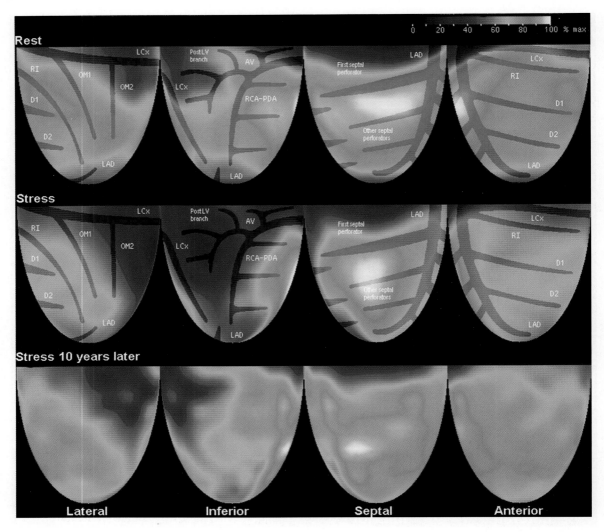

Fig. 2.12 Effect of intense medical therapy on progression of non-revascularized CAD. Rest perfusion image (*upper row*) shows a small transmural scar in the distribution of the distal LCx that is more severe and larger after dipyridamole stress (*middle row*). Follow-up PET (*lower row*) after 10 years of intense medical therapy shows that the stress induced perfusion defect is markedly smaller

lifestyle regimen maintaining 10% fat food, lean weight, regular exercise, Lipitor 5 mg, and Niaspan 1,000 mg daily achieving total cholesterol of 154 mg/dl, triglycerides 81 mg/dl, LDL 75 mg/dl, and HDL 63 mg/dl for the next 10 years. On the follow-up PET at 10 years, the stress induced perfusion defect is markedly smaller, essentially the same size as the small transmural scar on the baseline resting image and the patient had no exertional angina. With a documented LCX occlusion, this improvement is due to extensive collateral

development with flow capacity that approaches that of the native artery under dipyridamole stress.

Since the first concept of viability, FDG imaging by PET has been the gold standard for myocardial viability assessment due to its proven value in predicting functional outcomes after revascularization [61, 64, 89, 90] and in risk assessment for those patients with viable myocardium who are treated conservatively [76, 82, 91]. This leading role for PET in assessing viability has continued into current literature with further advances in PET imaging in comparison to other advanced imaging technologies. In a recent study, FDG PET had positive predictive value of 86%, negative predictive value of 100%, and diagnostic accuracy of 90% for recovery of LV function after revascularization [92]. Studies assessing viability with dobutamine MRI studies have reported comparable diagnostic accuracy but may have used a more selected study population [92]. The clinical value of FDG viability imaging can be further increased by gated FDG studies. The presence of LVEF < 25%, an end-diastolic LV volume > 260 ml, and of perfusion-mismatch pattern on gated FDG PET reliably identifies a patient population at highest risk with incremental value over viability information alone [93].

Essential Conditions for FDG PET Imaging

Clinical interpretation of FDG PET images depends on whether the patient is in a fasting or fed condition. Under fasting conditions, normal myocardium will metabolize fatty acids and will not uptake FDG; ischemic viable myocardium will take up FDG and create a positive image of the ischemic viable area. However, with fasting, areas of no FDG uptake can represent either normal myocardium or scar, thereby preventing a definitive clinical interpretation. After a carbohydrate meal or following a glucose load, both normal and ischemic viable myocardium will take up FDG and create a positive image of normal and ischemic viable myocardium; areas of scar will not take up FDG and therefore produce an image defect. Accordingly, PET protocols may vary depending upon the clinical or research question [94]. However, the standard clinical protocol now is to perform FDG PET imaging after a carbohydrate meal, with glucose loading before the scan and for diabetics a low fixed intravenous dose of insulin to reduce fatty acids levels and to assure myocardial uptake of FDG in all areas of viable myocardium except scar. Additional protocol details can be obtained from the American Society for Nuclear Cardiology and Society of Nuclear Medicine guidelines [95].

For assessing viability of a non-contractile myocardial region, the non-fasting, fed patient is given an oral glucose load and resting perfusion images are obtained with ^{13}N-ammonia or ^{82}Rb prior to FDG in order to identify hypoperfused areas. FDG is then injected intravenously and 45 min later, resting images are again obtained. Normal and ischemic viable myocardium will take up FDG but scar tissue will not. A perfusion–metabolism mismatch (low perfusion, FDG uptake) in poorly contracting segments identifies hibernating myocardium. Normal resting perfusion and FDG uptake with poor contraction identifies stunned myocardium. Areas with severe defects of both perfusion and FDG images (low or no FDG uptake) represent scarred or necrotic myocardium. Areas of normal perfusion and no FDG uptake with normal contraction indicate normal preferential uptake of fatty acids rather than FDG in the presence of adequate oxygen supply. A common variation of this protocol determines both flow limiting stenoses and viability by sequential rest perfusion imaging followed by dipyridamole or adenosine stress perfusion imaging followed by resting FDG imaging.

If the clinical question is whether the viable myocardium is normally oxygenated or metabolically ischemic due to a coronary artery stenosis, imaging is done with the patient in fasting state and with exercise stress. Under such circumstances, ischemic myocardium will take up FDG, whereas normal or scarred myocardium will not. A resting perfusion scan (with ^{13}N-ammonia or ^{82}Rb) is obtained first, followed by exercise carried out on a treadmill with reinjection of the perfusion tracer at peak stress, which is maintained for another 45–60 s, followed by stress imaging. While the patient is recovering after exercise, FDG is injected and 45 min later, FDG imaging is started. Transiently ischemic myocardium during stress will continue to take up FDG for hours after the stress induced ischemia has resolved due to the induction of metabolic pathways for FDG uptake by transient ischemia. An area with normal perfusion at rest, but with a stress induced perfusion defect and FDG uptake is metabolically ischemic due to a severe flow-limiting coronary stenosis. An area with normal perfusion at rest, a stress induced perfusion defect, and no FDG uptake has a mild/moderate flow-limiting stenosis that is not severe enough to cause metabolic ischemia. An area with severe rest and stress perfusion defects and no FDG uptake represents myocardial scar. However, this fasting protocol for assessing metabolic ischemia is seldom used clinically, since a flow-limiting stenosis causing a significant stress-induced perfusion abnormality is commonly considered adequate grounds for revascularization.

There are limitations in the use of FDG for viability assessment. Normal myocardium (normal perfusion and normal metabolism) in diabetics may not take up FDG due to insulin resistance associated with elevated free fatty acids in blood. Consequently, there is no FDG uptake anywhere in the heart and the study is uninterpretable. However, giving insulin intravenously at the time of glucose loading enhances myocardial uptake, reduces free fatty acids in blood, and provides diagnostic images.

With appropriate attention to patient preparation, FDG PET in diabetics for assessing viability reportedly has high sensitivity (92%) and specificity (85%) [96]. A perfusion FDG mismatch on PET in diabetic patients reliably identifies high risk for cardiac death with medical treatment compared to revascularization [97].

Limitations of FDG Imaging

^{18}F-fluoro-2-deoxyglucose imaging in fasting, resting state should not be performed in the early stages of evolving or recovery from an acute myocardial infarction. In such circumstances, FDG uptake is highly variable, sufficient to preclude interpretation, with intense uptake in necrotic areas due to uptake of FDG by inflammatory cells giving a false positive diagnosis of viable tissue. Moreover, FDG uptake may not parallel glucose metabolism [98, 99], with regional heterogeneity of uptake related to blood concentrations of glucose, insulin, fatty acids, catecholamines, and beta-blockers. Lastly, FDG studies with perfusion and metabolic imaging usually require up to 3 h, thereby limiting the patient volume and revenues.

Alternatives to FDG for detecting viable myocardium are based on myocardial leak of creatine phosphokinase, inosine, inorganic phosphate [100–103] due to impaired cell membrane function induced by ischemia and/or necrosis. Therefore, the use of a potassium analogue reflecting myocardial cellular membrane function and the myocardial potassium space represents an alternative for a quantitative assessment of viability and infarction size. ^{201}Tl is a potassium analogue for SPECT assessment of perfusion and myocardial viability that has well-documented value both experimentally and clinically. However, SPECT is limited by attenuation artifacts and depth-dependent poor resolution compared to PET.

^{82}Rb is a potassium analogue from commercially available ^{82}Strontium generators. After intravenous injection, ^{82}Rb is rapidly extracted and trapped in the potassium space of normal/viable myocardium but leaks out of necrotic cells as determined by histochemical methods leaving a perfusion defect [104]. The size of myocardial infarction determined by the size of the defect in ^{82}Rb uptake on rest images equals the size of myocardial infarction as detected by FDG imaging [67, 79]. In contrast to FDG, one ^{82}Rb viability study will take 1 h to complete, allowing higher volume per unit of time.

Thus, viable or necrotic myocardium can be identified by either by measures of glucose metabolism (FDG) with PET imaging or cell membrane integrity using potassium analogs such as ^{201}Tl with SPECT imaging or ^{82}Rb with PET imaging. However, the ability of ^{82}Rb washout between early and late resting imaging to reliably predict presence of viable myocardium as compared to identification of a perfusion–metabolism mismatch by FDG has been challenged in a recent study [105]. The authors reported poor specificity of ^{82}Rb washout for identifying areas of viable myocardium. On the other hand, their methodology for quantifying ^{82}Rb washout is open to question, since loss of the potassium space with corresponding defects on myocardial images of potassium analogs has been documented experimentally and clinically as a marker of necrotic or scarred myocardium.

The value of SPECT viability imaging with ^{201}Tl is well established clinically with overall 70–75% accuracy for predicting recovery of LV function compared to PET [28, 29, 61, 89]. For MIBI, predictive accuracy decreases to 64% compared to PET [106, 107]. Some of these discrepancies are explained by frequent inferior wall attenuation artifacts encountered with SPECT [4, 108]. The randomized trial CHRISTMAS (Carvedilol Hibernating Reversible Ischemia) demonstrated that SPECT MIBI predicted LV functional recovery in patients receiving carvedilol [109] with LVEF improving by 3.8%, more in those patients with hibernating myocardium by SPECT compared to those with no viable tissue. Whether such a small change is relevant for improved quality of life and prolonged survival was not determined. Larger controlled clinical trials are necessary to evaluate the role of revascularization in managing patients with heart failure due to ischemic heart disease [5]. The ongoing STITCH trial (Surgical Treatment for Ischemic Heart Failure) may provide an answer by randomizing patients with ischemic cardiomyopathy to medical therapy or CAB surgery based on SPECT imaging.

The value of PET for predicting clinical outcomes is complex, since the relevant end points include LV function, symptoms, reduced hospitalizations, and mortality. The utility of PET for assessing viability will vary for each of these endpoints. Most studies on changes in LV function as related to myocardial viability imaging have been performed in patients with moderately impaired systolic performance without quantifying the size of the viable myocardium or scar. In these studies the positive predictive accuracy decreases significantly in patients with more severe LV dysfunction (LVEF <30–35%) [110]. In patients with severe LV dysfunction, quantification of the amount of viable myocardium as more than 31% of the left ventricle accurately predicts improvement in LVEF after revascularization [111, 112].

Clinically significant improvement of symptoms and reduction of repeat hospitalizations are also more accurately predicted in those patients with hibernating myocardium comprising more than 18% of the whole heart, particularly in the LAD coronary artery territory [75, 113]. Patients with large areas of hibernating myocardium will have a poor outcome if treated conservatively with medical therapy compared to revascularization [79, 113]. For these patients with large zones at risk, revascularization is associated with improved outcomes, irrespective of the method used for assessing viability, including SPECT, PET, or dobutamine echocardiography as reported by meta-analysis [88].

The value of PET for predicting contractile function after revascularization depends on whether perfusion or metabolic imaging is performed, or both. For perfusion imaging alone, if regional blood flow is preserved to more than 50% of normal, contractile dysfunction will likely recover with an average positive and negative predictive value of 63% (range 45–78% and 45–100%, respectively) [114]. Compared to perfusion imaging alone, PET metabolic imaging of ^{11}C-acetate predicts functional recovery with a higher average positive predictive value of 72% and average negative predictive value of 76% (range 62–88% and 65–89%, respectively) [114].

Meta-analysis of perfusion—metabolism PET imaging for viability may not take into account the essential variables outlined above, differences in patient selection, or potential technical problems causing imaging artifacts [115]. Consequently, even when both measures of perfusion and metabolism are evaluated, the average positive predictive accuracy in predicting myocardial functional recovery after revascularization has a wide range of 52–100% with an average of 76%. The average negative predictive accuracy has an equally wide range of 67–100% with an average of 82% [114]. However, with optimal choice of patients, attention to medical and technical details with quantitative extent of viable myocardium, the accuracy of selecting patients for revascularization procedures approaches the upper end of the these ranges—over 90%.

FDG PET and ^{201}Tl SPECT may be particularly useful in the future for following replacement of infarcted myocardium using intracoronary injections of progenitor cells. In a small series of patients, this approach demonstrated a significant increase in myocardial viability and perfusion [116].

Molecular Imaging

From the original applications in coronary perfusion, cell membrane integrity, and cellular metabolism, nuclear medicine is evolving toward in vivo imaging of vasoreceptor functions and gene expression in early and advanced coronary artery disease [117, 118] including end stages such as heart failure. A major development of cardiac molecular biology involves transfer of genetic information from DNA to RNA by *transcription* and subsequent protein synthesis based on RNA template by *translation*. Various molecular biology techniques allow manipulation of both DNA and RNA, identification of therapeutic and reporter genes, molecular probes, and target peptides.

Gene therapy represents an area of great research interest due to potential expression of local therapeutic factors specific for the disease process with a parallel need for clinical methods of imaging these localized processes [119] using SPECT, PET, and MRI. Such targeted imaging requires several fundamental interacting elements: (i) a specific molecular *probe,* (ii) a *target* peptide for either a direct or indirect imaging strategy [120], and (iii) adequate *imaging characteristics* such as target size, stability and specificity of radionuclide localization, signal to noise, blood pool clearance, and radionuclides availability.

Direct methods use radiolabeled monoclonal antibodies (molecular probes) directed against cell surface antigens and receptors, or specific enzymes [120]. Cardiac applications of these techniques have been primarily designed to image alpha and beta adrenergic or muscarinic receptors [121] and drug pharmacokinetics including receptor binding [122].

Single photon emission tomography of ^{123}I-meta-iodobenzylguanidine (MIBG) images presynaptic sympathetic innervation of the heart. MIBG has a molecular structure similar to norepinephrine and is therefore taken up and stored in nerve presynaptic sympathetic endings [123]. In heart failure patients, low myocardial MIBG uptake combined with poor LV systolic performance (LVEF < 40%) [124, 125] and an accelerated MIBG washout rate [126] are independent predictors of mortality. For these patients, effects of drug therapy can be monitored using MIBG SPECT, including prediction of response to beta blockers [127, 128]. MIBG uptake is significantly reduced in areas of myocardial ischemia or infarction [129, 130], with the area of post infarct denervation being larger than the infarct related size of perfusion defects obtained with ^{201}Tl. Denervation of the viable area of myocardium around a scar contributes to increased vulnerability to ventricular arrhythmias [131].

Of particular interest for early detection of coronary artery disease is the observation that MIBG washout rate correlates inversely with the severity of coronary stenoses, suggesting that adrenergic function may be impaired prior to developing flow limiting stenoses [132]. Imaging the sympathetic system may be important for transplanted hearts. While the cardiac allograft is initially completely denervated, MIBG SPECT studies have demonstrated reinnervation as early as 1 year after transplantation, a process that may be impaired by graft vasculopathy [133].

Positron emission tomography offers substantial advantages over SPECT in imaging cardiac neurotransmission, primarily due to absolute quantification of radionuclide uptake as the basis for calculating receptor density, or drug-receptor interaction for specific myocardial regions of interest. Multiple tracers are available for PET imaging of the sympathetic system, using either radiolabeled catecholamines or cathecolamine analogues [134]. Most frequently used PET tracers are ^{11}Carbon-meta-hydroxiephedrine (HED) and ^{18}Fluorine-flurodopamine for studying ischemic heart disease [135, 136].

A reduction of HED uptake in patients with moderate heart failure is a predictor of poor outcome, a finding consistent with SPECT MIBG studies [137]. HED PET imaging demonstrates reinnervation of the transplanted heart [138] paralleling recovery of primarily fatty acids metabolism after an initial metabolic shift from fatty acids to glucose utilization associated with myocardial denervation [139].

Indirect imaging strategies such as reporter gene imaging [120] are more complex. This method involves delivery of a reporter gene to the target tissue via a viral or non-viral vector. The DNA of the reporter gene is transcribed to RNA with a reporter gene product generated via translation. The reporter gene product interacts with a reporter probe, leading to amplification of probe signal that may be imaged by PET, thereby localizing the reporter gene expression site and potentially the strength of expression [120].

Positron emission tomography reporter gene imaging may be particularly important for assessing angiogenic gene therapy in ischemic heart disease [140]. Hypoxia resulting from ischemia is the main stimulus for naturally occurring angiogenesis and collateral formation that provides blood flow to ischemic tissue [141]. Angiogenesis is mediated by a variety of factors, one of which is the vascular endothelial growth factor (VEGF), with ^{111}Indium labeled VEGF having high uptake in ischemic tissue [142]. Several clinical trials of coronary angiogenesis have been reported, some of which used MPI as an endpoint [143, 144]. Other trials used reporter gene imaging by linking a therapeutic gene to a reporter gene that is imaged by PET. Initial results of this approach have been reported using VEGF genes [145], recombinant human immunosuppresive cytokine interleukin-10 with intracoronary delivery [146], or other vectors with direct intramyocardial injection [147, 148].

Another approach images the expression of survival genes in hibernating myocardium with upregulation of anti-apoptosis and cytoprotective proteins as well as of growth factors—including VEGF [149]. The findings suggest a gene program for preventing cell death under conditions of prolonged ischemia. This study demonstrates the potential of PET gene imaging to evaluate hibernating or stunned viable myocardium or to monitor the effects of therapy aimed to enhance genetic survival mechanisms.

Molecular imaging may potentially address not only the pathophysiology of ischemia but also vascular inflammation causing rupture of atherosclerotic plaques before major ischemic events. Initial approaches have used imaging of [111]Indium radiolabeled monocytes [150], upregulated metalloproteinases [151], and imaging of apoptosis in atherosclerotic lesions [152]. However, none have evolved into clinically useful tests.

References

1. Bonow RO. The hibernating myocardium: implications for management of congestive heart failure. Am J Cardiol 1995; 75:17A–25A
2. Bonow RO. Functional evaluation of patients with coronary artery disease: selection of appropriate pharmacologic agents and imaging modalities. Eur Heart J 1995; 16 Suppl M:11–16
3. Dilsizian V, Bonow RO, Cannon RO, III, Tracy CM, Vitale DF, McIntosh CL et al. The effect of coronary artery bypass grafting on left ventricular systolic function at rest: evidence for preoperative subclinical myocardial ischemia. Am J Cardiol 1988; 61:1248–1254
4. Dilsizian V, Perrone-Filardi P, Arrighi JA, Bacharach SL, Quyyumi AA, Freedman NM et al. Concordance and discordance between stress-redistribution-reinjection and rest-redistribution thallium imaging for assessing viable myocardium. Comparison with metabolic activity by positron emission tomography. Circulation 1993; 88:941–952
5. Holly TA, Bonow RO. Assessment of myocardial viability with thallium-201 and technetium-based agents. In:

Zaret BL, Beller G. Clinical nuclear cardiology state of the art and future directions. 3rd ed. Philadelphia: Mosby, pp 503–517, 2005
6. Heyndrickx GR, Millard RW, McRitchie RJ, Maroko PR, Vatner SF. Regional myocardial functional and electrophysiological alterations after brief coronary artery occlusion in conscious dogs. J Clin Invest 1975; 56:978–985
7. Braunwald E, Kloner RA. The stunned myocardium: prolonged, postischemic ventricular dysfunction. Circulation 1982; 66:1146–1149
8. Diamond GA, Forrester JS, deLuz PL, Wyatt HL, Swan HJ. Post-extrasystolic potentiation of ischemic myocardium by atrial stimulation. Am Heart J 1978; 95:204–209
9. Rahimtoola SH. A perspective on the three large multicenter randomized clinical trials of coronary bypass surgery for chronic stable angina. Circulation 1985; 72:V123–V135
10. Murry CE, Jennings RB, Reimer KA. Preconditioning with ischemia: a delay of lethal cell injury in ischemic myocardium. Circulation 1986; 74:1124–1136
11. Taegtmeyer H. Metabolism—the lost child of cardiology. J Am Coll Cardiol 2000; 36:1386–1388
12. Gould KL. Assessing myocardial viability. In: Gould KL. Coronary artery stenosis and reversing atherosclerosis. 2nd ed. London: Arnold, pp 329–357, 1999
13. Akins CW, Pohost GM, Desanctis RW, Block PC. Selection of angina-free patients with severe left ventricular dysfunction for myocardial revascularization. Am J Cardiol 1980; 46:695–700
14. Johnson NP, Gould KL. Clinical evaluation of a new concept: resting myocardial perfusion heterogeneity quantified by markovian analysis of PET identifies coronary microvascular dysfunction and early atherosclerosis in 1,034 subjects. J Nucl Med 2005; 46:1427–1437
15. Ross J, Jr. Myocardial perfusion-contraction matching. Implications for coronary heart disease and hibernation. Circulation 1991; 83:1076–1083
16. Gould KL, Lipscomb K. Effects of coronary stenoses on coronary flow reserve and resistance. Am J Cardiol 1974; 34:48–55
17. Gould KL, Lipscomb K, Hamilton GW. Physiologic basis for assessing critical coronary stenosis. Instantaneous flow response and regional distribution during coronary hyperemia as measures of coronary flow reserve. Am J Cardiol 1974; 33:87–94
18. Gould KL, Schelbert HR, Phelps ME, Hoffman EJ. Noninvasive assessment of coronary stenoses with myocardial perfusion imaging during pharmacologic coronary vasodilatation. V. Detection of 47 percent diameter coronary stenosis with intravenous nitrogen-13 ammonia and emission-computed tomography in intact dogs. Am J Cardiol 1979; 43:200–208
19. Gould KL. Collapsing coronary stenosis – a starling resistor. Int J Cardiol 1982; 2:39–42
20. Gould KL, Kelley KO. Physiological significance of coronary flow velocity and changing stenosis geometry during coronary vasodilation in awake dogs. Circ Res 1982; 50:695–704
21. Kirkeeide RL, Gould KL, Parsel L. Assessment of coronary stenoses by myocardial perfusion imaging during

pharmacologic coronary vasodilation. VII. Validation of coronary flow reserve as a single integrated functional measure of stenosis severity reflecting all its geometric dimensions. J Am Coll Cardiol 1986; 7:103–113

22. Gould KL, Kirkeeide RL, Buchi M. Coronary flow reserve as a physiologic measure of stenosis severity. J Am Coll Cardiol 1990; 15:459–474

23. Gould KL. Detecting and assessing severity of coronary artery disease in humans. Cardiovasc Intervent Radiol 1990; 13:5–13

24. Gould KL. Coronary artery stenosis and reversing atherosclerosis. 2nd ed. London: Arnold; 1999

25. Nakagawa Y, Nakagawa K, Sdringola S, Mullani N, Gould KL. A precise, three-dimensional atlas of myocardial perfusion correlated with coronary arteriographic anatomy. J Nucl Cardiol 2001; 8:580–590

26. Rozanski A, Berman DS, Gray R, Levy R, Raymond M, Maddahi J et al. Use of thallium-201 redistribution scintigraphy in the preoperative differentiation of reversible and nonreversible myocardial asynergy. Circulation 1981;64:936–944

27. Iskandrian AS, Hakki AH, Kane SA, Goel IP, Mundth ED, Hakki AH et al. Rest and redistribution thallium-201 myocardial scintigraphy to predict improvement in left ventricular function after coronary arterial bypass grafting. Am J Cardiol 1983; 51:1312–1316

28. Cloninger KG, DePuey EG, Garcia EV, Roubin GS, Robbins WL, Nody A et al. Incomplete redistribution in delayed thallium-201 single photon emission computed tomographic (SPECT) images: an overestimation of myocardial scarring. J Am Coll Cardiol 1988; 12:955–963

29. Brunken RC, Kottou S, Nienaber CA, Schwaiger M, Ratib OM, Phelps ME et al. PET detection of viable tissue in myocardial segments with persistent defects at Tl-201 SPECT. Radiology 1989; 172:65–73

30. Tamaki N, Yonekura Y, Yamashita K, Senda M, Saji H, Hashimoto T et al. Relation of left ventricular perfusion and wall motion with metabolic activity in persistent defects on thallium-201 tomography in healed myocardial infarction. Am J Cardiol 1988; 62:202–208

31. Tamaki N, Ohtani H, Yamashita K, Magata Y, Yonekura Y, Nohara R et al. Metabolic activity in the areas of new fill-in after thallium-201 reinjection: comparison with positron emission tomography using fluorine-18-deoxyglucose. J Nucl Med 1991; 32:673–678

32. Gould KL, Goldstein RA, Mullani NA, Kirkeeide RL, Wong WH, Tewson TJ et al. Noninvasive assessment of coronary stenoses by myocardial perfusion imaging during pharmacologic coronary vasodilation. VIII. Clinical feasibility of positron cardiac imaging without a cyclotron using generator-produced rubidium-82. J Am Coll Cardiol 1986; 7:775–789

33. Dilsizian V, Rocco TP, Freedman NM, Leon MB, Bonow RO. Enhanced detection of ischemic but viable myocardium by the reinjection of thallium after stress-redistribution imaging. N Engl J Med 1990; 323:141–146

34. Sinusas AJ, Watson DD, Cannon JM, Jr., Beller GA. Effect of ischemia and postischemic dysfunction on myocardial uptake of technetium-99m-labeled methoxyisobutyl isonitrile and thallium-201. J Am Coll Cardiol 1989; 14:1785–1793

35. Beanlands RS, Dawood F, Wen WH, McLaughlin PR, Butany J, D'Amati G et al. Are the kinetics of technetium-99m methoxyisobutyl isonitrile affected by cell metabolism and viability? Circulation 1990; 82:1802–1814

36. Christian TF, Behrenbeck T, Pellikka PA, Huber KC, Chesebro JH, Gibbons RJ. Mismatch of left ventricular function and infarct size demonstrated by technetium-99m isonitrile imaging after reperfusion therapy for acute myocardial infarction: identification of myocardial stunning and hyperkinesia. J Am Coll Cardiol 1990; 16:1632–1638

37. Levine MG, McGill CC, Ahlberg AW, White MP, Giri S, Shareef B et al. Functional assessment with electrocardiographic gated single-photon emission computed tomography improves the ability of technetium-99m sestamibi myocardial perfusion imaging to predict myocardial viability in patients undergoing revascularization. Am J Cardiol 1999; 83:1–5

38. He ZX, Verani MS. Evaluation of myocardial viability by myocardial perfusion imaging: should nitrates be used? J Nucl Cardiol 1998; 5:527–532

39. Berman DS, Kiat H, Friedman JD, Wang FP, van TK, Matzer L et al. Separate acquisition rest thallium-201/stress technetium-99m sestamibi dual-isotope myocardial perfusion single-photon emission computed tomography: a clinical validation study. J Am Coll Cardiol 1993; 22:1455–1464

40. Heo J, Wolmer I, Kegel J, Iskandrian AS. Sequential dual-isotope SPECT imaging with thallium-201 and technetium-99m-sestamibi. J Nucl Med 1994; 35:549–553

41. Fukuzawa S, Inagaki M, Morooka S, Inoue T, Matsumoto Y, Yokoyama K et al. Evaluation of myocardial viability using sequential dual-isotope single photon emission tomography imaging with rest TI-201/stress Tc-99m tetrofosmin in the prediction of wall motion recovery after revascularization. Jpn Circ J 1997; 61:481–487

42. Tamaki N, Yonekura Y, Yamashita K, Saji H, Magata Y, Senda M et al. Positron emission tomography using fluorine-18 deoxyglucose in evaluation of coronary artery bypass grafting. Am J Cardiol 1989; 64:860–865

43. Gerber BL, Vanoverschelde JL, Bol A, Michel C, Labar D, Wijns W et al. Myocardial blood flow, glucose uptake, and recruitment of inotropic reserve in chronic left ventricular ischemic dysfunction. Implications for the pathophysiology of chronic myocardial hibernation. Circulation 1996; 94:651–659

44. Maki M, Luotolahti M, Nuutila P, Iida H, Voipio-Pulkki LM, Ruotsalainen U et al. Glucose uptake in the chronically dysfunctional but viable myocardium. Circulation 1996; 93:1658–1666

45. Fallavollita JA, Canty JM, Jr. Differential 18F-2-deoxyglucose uptake in viable dysfunctional myocardium with normal resting perfusion: evidence for chronic stunning in pigs. Circulation 1999; 99:2798–2805

46. Schelbert HR. Are the irreversible perfusion defects on myocardial thallium scans really irreversible? Eur Heart J 1988; 9 Suppl F:23–28

47. Camici P, Ferrannini E, Opie LH. Myocardial metabolism in ischemic heart disease: basic principles and application to imaging by positron emission tomography. Prog Cardiovasc Dis 1989; 32:217–238

48. Tamaki N, Yonekura Y, Yamashita K, Saji H, Magata Y, Senda M et al. Positron emission tomography using fluorine-18 deoxyglucose in evaluation of coronary artery bypass grafting. Am J Cardiol 1989; 64:860–865

49. Gropler RJ, Geltman EM, Sampathkumaran K, Perez JE, Schechtman KB, Conversano A et al. Comparison of carbon-11-acetate with fluorine-18-fluorodeoxyglucose for delineating viable myocardium by positron emission tomography. J Am Coll Cardiol 1993; 22:1587–1597

50. Gropler RJ, Geltman EM, Sampathkumaran K, Perez JE, Moerlein SM, Sobel BE et al. Functional recovery after coronary revascularization for chronic coronary artery disease is dependent on maintenance of oxidative metabolism. J Am Coll Cardiol 1992; 20:569–577

51. Buxton DB, Nienaber CA, Luxen A, Ratib O, Hansen H, Phelps ME et al. Noninvasive quantitation of regional myocardial oxygen consumption in vivo with [1-11C]acetate and dynamic positron emission tomography. Circulation 1989; 79:134–142

52. Armbrecht JJ, Buxton DB, Schelbert HR. Validation of [1-11C]acetate as a tracer for noninvasive assessment of oxidative metabolism with positron emission tomography in normal, ischemic, postischemic, and hyperemic canine myocardium. Circulation 1990; 81:1594–1605

53. Ter-Pogossian MM, Klein MS, Markham J, Roberts R, Sobel BE. Regional assessment of myocardial metabolic integrity in vivo by positron-emission tomography with 11C-labeled palmitate. Circulation 1980; 61:242–255

54. Geltman EM, Biello D, Welch MJ, Ter-Pogossian MM, Roberts R, Sobel BE. Characterization of nontransmural myocardial infarction by positron-emission tomography. Circulation 1982; 65:747–755

55. Sobel BE, Geltman EM, Tiefenbrunn AJ, Jaffe AS, Spadaro JJ, Jr., Ter-Pogossian MM et al. Improvement of regional myocardial metabolism after coronary thrombolysis induced with tissue-type plasminogen activator or streptokinase. Circulation 1984; 69:983–990

56. Gould KL. Coronary artery stenosis and reversing atherosclerosis. 2nd ed. London: Arnold; 1999

57. Merhige ME, Ekas R, Mossberg K, Taegtmeyer H, Gould KL. Catecholamine stimulation, substrate competition, and myocardial glucose uptake in conscious dogs assessed with positron emission tomography. Circ Res 1987; 61:II124–II129

58. Rhodes CG, Camici PG, Taegtmeyer H, Doenst T. Variability of the lumped constant for [18F]2-deoxy-2-fluoroglucose and the experimental isolated rat heart model: clinical perspectives for the measurement of myocardial tissue viability in humans. Circulation 1999; 99:1275–1276

59. Doenst T, Holden JE, Taegtmeyer H. Limitations to the assessment of reperfusion injury with radiolabeled 2-deoxyglucose. Circulation 1999; 99:1646–1647

60. Doenst T, Taegtmeyer H. Profound underestimation of glucose uptake by [18F]2-deoxy-2-fluoroglucose in reperfused rat heart muscle. Circulation 1998; 97:2454–2462

61. Tillisch J, Brunken R, Marshall R, Schwaiger M, Mandelkern M, Phelps M et al. Reversibility of cardiac wall-motion abnormalities predicted by positron tomography. N Engl J Med 1986; 314:884–888

62. Tamaki N, Yonekura Y, Yamashita K, Saji H, Magata Y, Senda M et al. Positron emission tomography using fluorine-18 deoxyglucose in evaluation of coronary artery bypass grafting. Am J Cardiol 1989; 64:860–865

63. Tamaki N, Yonekura Y, Yamashita K, Senda M, Saji H, Konishi Y et al. Value of rest-stress myocardial positron tomography using nitrogen-13 ammonia for the preoperative prediction of reversible asynergy. J Nucl Med 1989; 30:1302–1310

64. Marwick TH, Nemec JJ, Lafont A, Salcedo EE, MacIntyre WJ. Prediction by postexercise fluoro-18 deoxyglucose positron emission tomography of improvement in exercise capacity after revascularization. Am J Cardiol 1992; 69:854–859

65. Di Carli MF, Prcevski P, Singh TP, Janisse J, Ager J, Muzik O et al. Myocardial blood flow, function, and metabolism in repetitive stunning. J Nucl Med 2000; 41:1227–1234

66. Gould KL. Quantification of coronary artery stenosis in vivo. Circ Res 1985; 57:341–353

67. Gould KL, Yoshida K, Hess MJ, Haynie M, Mullani N, Smalling RW. Myocardial metabolism of fluorodeoxyglucose compared to cell membrane integrity for the potassium analogue rubidium-82 for assessing infarct size in man by PET. J Nucl Med 1991; 32:1–9

68. Ritchie JL, Bateman TM, Bonow RO, Crawford MH, Gibbons RJ, Hall RJ et al. Guidelines for clinical use of cardiac radionuclide imaging. Report of the American College of Cardiology/American Heart Association Task Force on Assessment of Diagnostic and Therapeutic Cardiovascular Procedures (Committee on Radionuclide Imaging), developed in collaboration with the American Society of Nuclear Cardiology. J Am Coll Cardiol 1995; 25:521–547

69. Brindis RG, Douglas PS, Hendel RC, Peterson ED, Wolk MJ, Allen JM et al. ACCF/ASNC appropriateness criteria for single-photon emission computed tomography myocardial perfusion imaging (SPECT MPI): a report of the American College of Cardiology Foundation Quality Strategic Directions Committee Appropriateness Criteria Working Group and the American Society of Nuclear Cardiology endorsed by the American Heart Association. J Am Coll Cardiol 2005; 46:1587–1605

70. Brown KA. Prognostic value of myocardial perfusion imaging: state of the art and new developments. J Nucl Cardiol 1996; 3:516–537

71. Brown KA, Heller GV, Landin RS, Shaw LJ, Beller GA, Pasquale MJ et al. Early dipyridamole (99m)Tc-sestamibi single photon emission computed tomographic imaging 2 to 4 days after acute myocardial infarction predicts in-hospital and postdischarge cardiac events: comparison with submaximal exercise imaging. Circulation 1999; 100:2060–2066

72. Kitsiou AN, Srinivasan G, Quyyumi AA, Summers RM, Bacharach SL, Dilsizian V. Stress-induced reversible and

mild-to-moderate irreversible thallium defects: are they equally accurate for predicting recovery of regional left ventricular function after revascularization? Circulation 1998; 98:501–508

73. Mori T, Minamiji K, Kurogane H, Ogawa K, Yoshida Y. Rest-injected thallium-201 imaging for assessing viability of severe asynergic regions. J Nucl Med 1991; 32:1718–1724

74. Cornel JH, Bax JJ, Elhendy A, Maat AP, Kimman GJ, Geleijnse ML et al. Biphasic response to dobutamine predicts improvement of global left ventricular function after surgical revascularization in patients with stable coronary artery disease: implications of time course of recovery on diagnostic accuracy. J Am Coll Cardiol 1998; 31:1002–1010

75. Di Carli MF, Asgarzadie F, Schelbert HR, Brunken RC, Laks H, Phelps ME et al. Quantitative relation between myocardial viability and improvement in heart failure symptoms after revascularization in patients with ischemic cardiomyopathy. Circulation 1995; 92:3436–3444

76. Tamaki N, Kawamoto M, Takahashi N, Yonekura Y, Magata Y, Nohara R et al. Prognostic value of an increase in fluorine-18 deoxyglucose uptake in patients with myocardial infarction: comparison with stress thallium imaging. J Am Coll Cardiol 1993; 22:1621–1627

77. Lee KS, Marwick TH, Cook SA, Go RT, Fix JS, James KB et al. Prognosis of patients with left ventricular dysfunction, with and without viable myocardium after myocardial infarction. Relative efficacy of medical therapy and revascularization. Circulation 1994; 90:2687–2694

78. Gould KL. Coronary artery stenosis and reversing atherosclerosis. 2nd ed. London: Arnold; 1999

79. Yoshida K, Gould KL. Quantitative relation of myocardial infarct size and myocardial viability by positron emission tomography to left ventricular ejection fraction and 3-year mortality with and without revascularization. J Am Coll Cardiol 1993; 22:984–997

80. Sdringola S, Nakagawa K, Nakagawa Y, Yusuf SW, Boccalandro F, Mullani N et al. Combined intense lifestyle and pharmacologic lipid treatment further reduce coronary events and myocardial perfusion abnormalities compared with usual-care cholesterol-lowering drugs in coronary artery disease. J Am Coll Cardiol 2003; 41:263–272

81. Rizvi AA, Velusamy M, Heller GV. Evaluation of myocardial viability. In: Heller GV, Hendel R. Nuclear cardiology practical applications. New York: McGraw Hill, Medical Pub. Division, pp 49–65, 2004

82. Di Carli MF, Davidson M, Little R, Khanna S, Mody FV, Brunken RC et al. Value of metabolic imaging with positron emission tomography for evaluating prognosis in patients with coronary artery disease and left ventricular dysfunction. Am J Cardiol 1994; 73:527–533

83. Eitzman D, al-Aouar Z, Kanter HL, vom DJ, Kirsh M, Deeb GM et al. Clinical outcome of patients with advanced coronary artery disease after viability studies with positron emission tomography. J Am Coll Cardiol 1992; 20:559–565

84. Ausma J, Cleutjens J, Thone F, Flameng W, Ramaekers F, Borgers M. Chronic hibernating myocardium: interstitial changes. Mol Cell Biochem 1995; 147:35–42

85. Bax JJ, Cornel JH, Visser FC, Fioretti PM, van LA, Reijs AE et al. Prediction of recovery of myocardial dysfunction after revascularization. Comparison of fluorine-18 fluorodeoxyglucose/thallium-201 SPECT, thallium-201 stress-reinjection SPECT and dobutamine echocardiography. J Am Coll Cardiol 1996; 28:558–564

86. Bax JJ, Wijns W, Cornel JH, Visser FC, Boersma E, Fioretti PM. Accuracy of currently available techniques for prediction of functional recovery after revascularization in patients with left ventricular dysfunction due to chronic coronary artery disease: comparison of pooled data. J Am Coll Cardiol 1997; 30:1451–1460

87. Vanoverschelde JLJ, Gerber B, Pasquet A, Melin JA. Physiologic and metabolic basis of myocardial viability imaging. In: Zaret BL, Beller G. Clinical nuclear cardiology state of the art and future directions. 3rd ed. Philadelphia: Mosby, pp 495–501, 2005

88. Allman KC, Shaw LJ, Hachamovitch R, Udelson JE. Myocardial viability testing and impact of revascularization on prognosis in patients with coronary artery disease and left ventricular dysfunction: a meta-analysis. J Am Coll Cardiol 2002; 39:1151–1158

89. Bonow RO, Dilsizian V, Cuocolo A, Bacharach SL. Identification of viable myocardium in patients with chronic coronary artery disease and left ventricular dysfunction. Comparison of thallium scintigraphy with reinjection and PET imaging with 18F-fluorodeoxyglucose. Circulation 1991; 83:26–37

90. Eitzman D, al-Aouar Z, Kanter HL, vom DJ, Kirsh M, Deeb GM et al. Clinical outcome of patients with advanced coronary artery disease after viability studies with positron emission tomography. J Am Coll Cardiol 1992; 20:559–565

91. Gould KL. Does positron emission tomography improve patient selection for coronary revascularization? J Am Coll Cardiol 1992; 20:566–568

92. Schmidt M, Voth E, Schneider CA, Theissen P, Wagner R, Baer FM et al. F-18-FDG uptake is a reliable predictory of functional recovery of akinetic but viable infarct regions as defined by magnetic resonance imaging before and after revascularization. Magn Reson Imaging 2004; 22:229–236

93. Santana CA, Shaw LJ, Garcia EV, Soler-Peter M, Candell-Riera J, Grossman GB et al. Incremental prognostic value of left ventricular function by myocardial ECG-gated FDG PET imaging in patients with ischemic cardiomyopathy. J Nucl Cardiol 2004; 11:542–550

94. Gould KL. Coronary artery stenosis and reversing atherosclerosis. 2nd ed. London: Arnold; 1999

95. Bacharach SL, Bax JJ, Case J, Delete D, Cordial KA, Martin WH et al. PET myocardial glucose metabolism and perfusion imaging: Part 1-Guidelines for data acquisition and patient preparation. J Nucl Cardiol 2003; 10:543–556

96. Schooner H, Campos R, Outtake T, Hoh CK, Moon DH, Czerny J et al. Blood flow-metabolism imaging with positron emission tomography in patients with diabetes mellitus for the assessment of reversible left ventricular contractile dysfunction. J Am Coll Cardiol 1999; 33:1328–1337

97. Sawada S, Hanoi O, Barclay J, Geiger S, Fain R, Foltz J et al. Usefulness of positron emission tomography in predicting long-term outcome in patients with diabetes mellitus and ischemic left ventricular dysfunction. Am J Cardiol 2005; 96:2–8

98. Marinara R, Bray M, Gamin R, Doenst T, Goodwin GW, Taegtmeyer H. Fundamental limitations of [18F]2-deoxy-2-fluoro-D-glucose for assessing myocardial glucose uptake. Circulation 1995; 91:2435–2444

99. Bolukoglu H, Goodwin GW, Guthrie PH, Carmical SG, Chen TM, Taegtmeyer H. Metabolic fate of glucose in reversible low-flow ischemia of the isolated working rat heart. Am J Physiol 1996; 270:H817–H826

100. de Jong JW, Goldstein S. Changes in coronary venous inosine concentration and myocardial wall thickening during regional ischemia in the pig. Circ Res 1974; 35:111–116

101. Opie LH, Thomas M, Owen P, Shulman G. Increased coronary venous inorganic phosphate concentrations during experimental myocardial ischemia. Am J Cardiol 1972; 30:503–513

102. Hill JL, Gettes LS. Effect of acute coronary artery occlusion on local myocardial extracellular K + activity in swine. Circulation 1980; 61:768–778

103. Nakaya H, Kimura S, Kanno M. Intracellular K + and Na + activities under hypoxia, acidosis, and no glucose in dog hearts. Am J Physiol 1985; 249:H1078–H1085

104. vom DJ, Muzik O, Wolfe ER, Jr., Allman C, Hutchins G, Schwaiger M. Myocardial rubidium-82 tissue kinetics assessed by dynamic positron emission tomography as a marker of myocardial cell membrane integrity and viability. Circulation 1996; 93:238–245

105. Stankewicz MA, Mansour CS, Eisner RL, Churchwell KB, Williams BR, Sigman SR et al. Myocardial viability assessment by PET: (82)Rb defect washout does not predict the results of metabolic-perfusion mismatch. J Nucl Med 2005; 46:1602–1609

106. Dilsizian V, Arrighi JA, Diodati JG, Quyyumi AA, Alavi K, Bacharach SL et al. Myocardial viability in patients with chronic coronary artery disease. Comparison of 99mTc-sestamibi with thallium reinjection and [18F]-fluorodeoxyglucose. Circulation 1994; 89:578–587

107. Sawada SG, Allman KC, Muzik O, Beanlands RS, Wolfe ER, Jr., Gross M et al. Positron emission tomography detects evidence of viability in rest technetium-99m sestamibi defects. J Am Coll Cardiol 1994; 23:92–98

108. Dilsizian V, Bonow RO. Current diagnostic techniques of assessing myocardial viability in patients with hibernating and stunned myocardium. Circulation 1993; 87:1–20

109. Cleland JG, Pennell DJ, Ray SG, Coats AJ, Macfarlane PW, Murray GD et al. Myocardial viability as a determinant of the ejection fraction response to carvedilol in patients with heart failure (CHRISTMAS trial): randomized controlled trial. Lancet 2003; 362:14–21

110. Di Carli MF, Maddahi J, Rokhsar S, Schelbert HR, Bianco-Batlles D, Brunken RC et al. Long-term survival of patients with coronary artery disease and left ventricular dysfunction: implications for the role of myocardial viability assessment in management decisions. J Thorac Cardiovasc Surg 1998; 116:997–1004

111. Bax JJ, Visser FC, Poldermans D, Elhendy A, Cornel JH, Boersma E et al. Relationship between preoperative viability and postoperative improvement in LVEF and heart failure symptoms. J Nucl Med 2001; 42:79–86

112. Di Carli MF, Hachamovitch R, Berman DS. The art and science of predicting postrevascularization improvement in left ventricular (LV) function in patients with severely depressed LV function. J Am Coll Cardiol 2002; 40:1744–1747

113. Rohatgi R, Epstein S, Henriquez J, Ababneh AA, Hickey KT, Pinsky D et al. Utility of positron emission tomography in predicting cardiac events and survival in patients with coronary artery disease and severe left ventricular dysfunction. Am J Cardiol 2001; 87:1096–1099, A6

114. Di Carli MF. Assessment of myocardial viability with positron emission tomography. In: Zaret BL, Beller G. Clinical nuclear cardiology state of the art and future directions. 3rd ed. Philadelphia: Mosby, pp 519–534, 2005

115. Loghin C, Sdringola S, Gould KL. Common artifacts in PET myocardial perfusion images due to attenuation-emission misregistration: clinical significance, causes, and solutions. J Nucl Med 2004; 45:1029–1039

116. Dobert N, Britten M, Assmus B, Berner U, Menzel C, Lehmann R et al. Transplantation of progenitor cells after reperfused acute myocardial infarction: evaluation of perfusion and myocardial viability with FDG-PET and thallium SPECT. Eur J Nucl Med Mol Imaging 2004; 31:1146–1151

117. Phelps ME. PET: the merging of biology and imaging into molecular imaging. J Nucl Med 2000; 41:661–681

118. Phelps ME. Inaugural article: positron emission tomography provides molecular imaging of biological processes. Proc Natl Acad Sci U S A 2000; 97:9226–9233

119. Herrero P, Gropler RJ. Imaging of myocardial metabolism. J Nucl Cardiol 2005; 12:345–358

120. Dobrucki LW, Sinusas AJ. Molecular imaging. A new approach to nuclear cardiology. Q J Nucl Med Mol Imaging 2005; 49:106–115

121. Raffel DM, Wieland DM. Assessment of cardiac sympathetic nerve integrity with positron emission tomography. Nucl Med Biol 2001; 28:541–559

122. Yoshinaga K, Chow BJ, deKemp RA, Thorn S, Ruddy TD, Davies RA et al. Application of cardiac molecular imaging using positron emission tomography in evaluation of drug and therapeutics for cardiovascular disorders. Curr Pharm Des 2005; 11:903–932

123. Knickmeier M, Matheja P, Wichter T, Schafers KP, Kies P, Breithardt G et al. Clinical evaluation of no-carrier-added meta-[123I]iodobenzylguanidine for myocardial scintigraphy. Eur J Nucl Med 2000; 27:302–307

124. Merlet P, Valette H, Dubois-Rande JL, Moyse D, Duboc D, Dove P et al. Prognostic value of cardiac metaiodobenzylguanidine imaging in patients with heart failure. J Nucl Med 1992; 33:471–477

125. Merlet P, Benvenuti C, Moyse D, Pouillart F, Dubois-Rande JL, Duval AM et al. Prognostic value of MIBG imaging in idiopathic dilated cardiomyopathy. J Nucl Med 1999; 40:917–923

126. Cohen-Solal A, Esanu Y, Logeart D, Pessione F, Dubois C, Dreyfus G et al. Cardiac metaiodobenzyl-guanidine uptake in patients with moderate chronic heart failure: relationship with peak oxygen uptake and prognosis. J Am Coll Cardiol 1999; 33:759–766

127. Suwa M, Otake Y, Moriguchi A, Ito T, Hirota Y, Kawamura K et al. Iodine-123 metaiodobenzylguani-dine myocardial scintigraphy for prediction of response to beta-blocker therapy in patients with dilated cardio-myopathy. Am Heart J 1997; 133:353–358

128. Gerson MC, Craft LL, McGuire N, Suresh DP, Abraham WT, Wagoner LE. Carvedilol improves left ventricular function in heart failure patients with idiopathic dilated cardiomyopathy and a wide range of sympathetic nervous system function as measured by iodine 123 metaiodoben-zylguanidine. J Nucl Cardiol 2002; 9:608–615

129. McGhie AI, Corbett JR, Akers MS, Kulkarni P, Sills MN, Kremers M et al. Regional cardiac adrenergic function using I-123 meta-iodobenzylguanidine tomo-graphic imaging after acute myocardial infarction. Am J Cardiol 1991; 67:236–242

130. Nishimura T, Oka H, Sago M, Matsuo T, Uehara T, Noda H et al. Serial assessment of denervated but viable myocardium following acute myocardial infarction in dogs using iodine-123 metaiodobenzylguanidine and thallium-201 chloride myocardial single photon emis-sion tomography. Eur J Nucl Med 1992; 19:25–29

131. Hartikainen J, Kuikka J, Mantysaari M, Lansimies E, Pyorala K. Sympathetic reinnervation after acute myocardial infarction. Am J Cardiol 1996; 77:5–9

132. Simula S, Vanninen E, Viitanen L, Kareinen A, Lehto S, Pajunen P et al. Cardiac adrenergic innervation is affected in asymptomatic subjects with very early stage of coronary artery disease. J Nucl Med 2002; 43:1–7

133. Estorch M, Camprecios M, Flotats A, Mari C, Berna L, Catafau AM et al. Sympathetic reinnervation of cardiac allografts evaluated by 123I-MIBG imaging. J Nucl Med 1999; 40:911–916

134. Bengel FM, Schwaiger M. Cardiac neurotransmission imaging; positron emission tomography. In: Zaret BL, Beller G. Clinical nuclear cardiology state of the art and future directions. 3rd ed. Philadelphia: Mosby, pp 593–607, 2005

135. Bengel FM, Permanetter B, Ungerer M, Nekolla SG, Schwaiger M. Relationship between altered sympa-thetic innervation, oxidative metabolism and contrac-tile function in the cardiomyopathic human heart; a non-invasive study using positron emission tomogra-phy. Eur Heart J 2001; 22:1594–1600

136. Goldstein DS, Eisenhofer G, Dunn BB, Armando I, Lenders J, Grossman E et al. Positron emission tomo-graphic imaging of cardiac sympathetic innervation using 6-[18F]fluorodopamine: initial findings in humans. J Am Coll Cardiol 1993; 22:1961–1971

137. Pietila M, Malminiemi K, Ukkonen H, Saraste M, Nagren K, Lehikoinen P et al. Reduced myocardial carbon-11 hydroxyephedrine retention is associated with poor prognosis in chronic heart failure. Eur J Nucl Med 2001; 28:373–376

138. Bengel FM, Ueberfuhr P, Hesse T, Schiepel N, Ziegler SI, Scholz S et al. Clinical determinants of ventricular sympathetic reinnervation after orthotopic heart transplantation. Circulation 2002; 106: 831–835

139. Bengel FM, Ueberfuhr P, Ziegler SI, Nekolla SG, Odaka K, Reichart B et al. Non-invasive assessment of the effect of cardiac sympathetic innervation on metabo-lism of the human heart. Eur J Nucl Med 2000; 27:1650–1657

140. Inubushi M, Tamaki N. Positron emission tomography reporter gene imaging in the myocardium: for monitor-ing of angiogenic gene therapy in ischemic heart disease. J Card Surg 2005; 20:S20–S24

141. Shweiki D, Itin A, Soffer D, Keshet E. Vascular endothe-lial growth factor induced by hypoxia may mediate hypoxia-initiated angiogenesis. Nature 1992; 359:843–845

142. Lu E, Wagner WR, Schellenberger U, Abraham JA, Klibanov AL, Woulfe SR et al. Targeted in vivo labeling of receptors for vascular endothelial growth factor: approach to identification of ischemic tissue. Circulation 2003; 108:97–103

143. Kleiman NS, Califf RM. Results from late-breaking clinical trials sessions at ACCIS 2000 and ACC 2000. American College of Cardiology. J Am Coll Cardiol 2000; 36:310–325

144. Henry TD, Annex BH, McKendall GR, Azrin MA, Lopez JJ, Giordano FJ et al. The VIVA trial: vascular endothelial growth factor in Ischemia for vascular angiogenesis. Circulation 2003; 107:1359–1365

145. Wu JC, Chen IY, Wang Y, Tseng JR, Chhabra A, Salek M et al. Molecular imaging of the kinetics of vascular endothelial growth factor gene expression in ischemic myocardium. Circulation 2004; 110:685–691

146. Sen L, Gambhir SS, Furukawa H, Stout DB, Linh LA, Laks H et al. Noninvasive imaging of ex vivo intracor-onarily delivered nonviral therapeutic transgene expres-sion in heart. Mol Ther 2005; 12:49–57

147. Bengel FM, Anton M, Richter T, Simoes MV, Haubner R, Henke J et al. Noninvasive imaging of transgene expression by use of positron emission tomography in a pig model of myocardial gene transfer. Circulation 2003; 108:2127–2133

148. Miyagawa M, Anton M, Haubner R, Simoes MV, Stadele C, Erhardt W et al. PET of cardiac transgene expression: comparison of 2 approaches based on herpesviral thymi-dine kinase reporter gene. J Nucl Med 2004; 45:1917–1923

149. Depre C, Kim SJ, John AS, Huang Y, Rimoldi OE, Pepper JR et al. Program of cell survival underlying human and experimental hibernating myocardium. Circ Res 2004; 95:433–440

150. Virgolini I, Muller C, Fitscha P, Chiba P, Sinzinger H. Radiolabeling autologous monocytes with 111-indium-oxine for reinjection in patients with atherosclerosis. Prog Clin Biol Res 1990; 355:271–280

151. Narula J, Verjans J, Zaret BL. Radionuclide approach to imaging of inflammation in atheroma for the detection of lesions vulnerable to rupture. In: Zaret BL, Beller G. Clinical nuclear cardiology state of the art and future directions. 3rd ed. Philadelphia: Mosby, pp 659–671, 2005

152. Kolodgie FD, Petrov A, Virmani R, Narula N, Verjans JW, Weber DK et al. Targeting of apoptotic macro-phages and experimental atheroma with radiolabeled annexin V: a technique with potential for noninvasive imaging of vulnerable plaque. Circulation 2003; 108:3134–3139

Chapter 3
Sudden Cardiac Death in Advanced Ischemic Heart Disease

Epidemiology, Etiology, and Defibrillator Therapy

Zian H. Tseng, Nitish Badhwar, and Teresa De Marco

Abstract Two thirds of the nearly half a million deaths per year in the United States due to sudden cardiac death (SCD) is attributed to coronary artery disease (CAD) and most commonly results from untreated ventricular tachyarrhythmias. Patients with ischemic cardiomyopathy and left ventricular dysfunction are at highest risk for SCD, but this still defines only a small subset of patients who will suffer SCD. Multiple lines of evidence now support the superiority of implantable cardioverter defibrillator (ICD) therapy over antiarrhythmic therapy for both primary and secondary prevention of SCD in advanced ischemic heart disease. Optimization of ICD therapy in advanced ischemic cardiomyopathy includes preventing right ventricular pacing as well as the use of highly effective anti-tachycardia pacing to reduce the number of shocks. While expensive, ICD therapy has been shown to compare favorably to the accepted standard of hemodialysis in cost effectiveness analyses.

Definition

Sudden cardiac death (SCD) is defined as a sudden, unexpected death from a cardiac cause less than an hour after the onset of cardiac symptoms. SCD most commonly results from cardiac arrest due to lethal ventricular tachyarrhythmias. SCD usually occurs in the setting of underlying structural heart disease, most commonly coronary artery disease (CAD). Cessation of cardiac function occurs, with or without resuscitation or spontaneous reversion. Patients who do not die after cardiac arrest are said to have experienced "aborted SCD," or to have survived a cardiac arrest.

Etiology and Epidemiology

Sudden cardiac death accounts for more deaths per year in the United States than stroke, lung cancer, breast cancer, and AIDS combined [1]. CAD is the underlying cause in 65–70% of all SCDs [2–4], with SCD occurring either as the initial manifestation of CAD or in those with a history of CAD and left ventricular dysfunction [5, 6]. Other forms of cardiac disease, such as hypertrophic cardiomyopathy and inherited sudden death syndromes (e.g., long QT syndrome, Brugada syndrome) are associated with SCD, but account for only a small portion of SCD patients. Approximately 60% of SCDs occur outside of a hospital setting [2]. First known arrhythmic events account for approximately 85–90% of SCDs while the remaining 10–15% are due to recurrent events [7]. From 1989 to 1998, the proportional rate of SCD increased as the underlying cause of all cardiac deaths [4].

There are differences in SCD rates among men and women as well as among different ethnic groups. Men account for approximately 75% of all SCDs [6] and, compared to women, have a 50% higher age-adjusted rate of SCD. Blacks have

Z.H. Tseng (✉)
Cardiac Electrophysiology Section, Department of Medicine, University of California, San Francisco, CA, USA
e-mail: zhtseng@medicine.ucsf.edu

R. Delgado, H.S. Arora (eds.), *Interventional Treatment of Advanced Ischemic Heart Disease*,
DOI 10.1007/978-1-84800-395-8_3, © Springer-Verlag London Limited 2009

higher age-adjusted mortality rates for SCD than whites, American Indians/Alaskan Natives, Hispanics, or Asian/Pacific Islanders [2].

Currently, the only clinically useful risk factors for SCD are the presence of CAD, previous myocardial infarction (MI), and depressed left ventricular (LV) function. While these factors account for the patients with the highest risk of SCD, they do not account for the majority of patients who have SCD (from the perspective of the total number of SCD patients) [5]. Most SCDs occur in the larger, lower risk subgroups, i.e., those who

would not have been included in ICD trials (Fig. 3.1).

Not all patients with MI and depressed LV function develop SCD or ventricular arrhythmias—it is estimated that 20–30% of patients with ischemic cardiomyopathy will develop SCD or ventricular arrhythmias [5, 8–10]. SCD rates vary with severity of heart failure (Fig. 3.2). The proportion of SCDs decreases with increasing severity of heart failure by NYHA functional class [11]. SCD accounts for the majority of deaths in those with NYHA II or III heart failure, while progressive heart failure

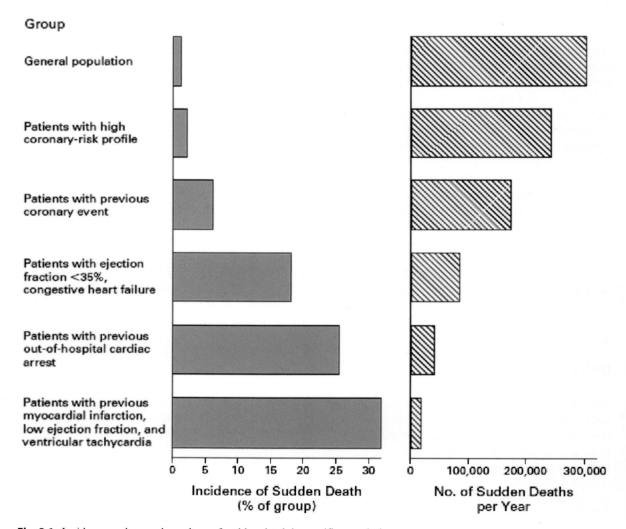

Fig. 3.1 Incidence and annual numbers of sudden death in specific populations

Fig. 3.2 Differences in mode of death with severity of heart failure

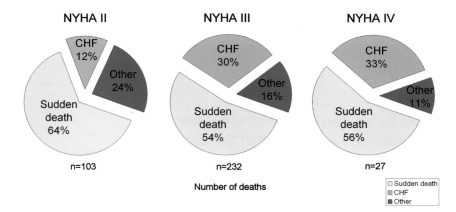

accounts for the majority of deaths in NYHA IV heart failure.

There is also evidence that genetics may play a role in the risk of SCD in the setting of CAD. Multifactorial analyses from two large epidemiologic studies have shown a familial risk of SCD that is independent of the risk of MI or CAD [12, 13]. The rate of SCD in the setting of CAD among first-degree relatives of SCD patients was almost 50% higher than those without a family history of SCD and was even higher when both sides of the family were affected.

Identification of Risk of Sudden Cardiac Death in Ischemic Cardiomyopathy

Current noninvasive risk stratification schemata for SCD in patients with CAD, including variables such as nonsustained ventricular tachycardia (VT), ejection fraction (EF), heart rate variability, baroreflex sensitivity, signal averaged electrocardiogram (SAECG), QT dispersion, and QRS duration, have not proven to be effective in identifying those patients at risk for SCD, even in the beta blocker era [14]. T wave alternans has been of recent interest for risk stratification [15, 16], but its value has not been proven by prospective validation. Even invasive electrophysiologic testing showed that patients with ischemic cardiomyopathy who were noninducible for ventricular tachyarrhythmias had essentially the same risk of SCD as those who were inducible [17]. Moreover, the positive predictive

accuracy of inducibility of VT has been relatively low in consecutive series of patients with recent MI [18, 19]. Therefore, at present, only LV dysfunction reliably defines "high-risk" for SCD in patients with ischemic cardiomyopathy.

Strategies for Prevention of Sudden Cardiac Death in Ischemic Cardiomyopathy

On the basis of two large randomized trials aimed at suppressing premature ventricular complexes after MI, so-called "warning arrhythmias," it was discovered that many common antiarrhythmic medications actually increase the risk of mortality [20, 21]. Amiodarone also has been shown to have no definitive effect on mortality in patients after an MI, including in the recent SCD-HeFT trial [22–24]. In fact, of all antiarrhythmic medications, only beta blockers have been clearly shown to prevent SCD after MI [25], particularly among those with depressed LV function [11].

Implantable cardioverter defibrillators, on the other hand, have demonstrated a remarkable effectiveness in prevention of SCD, with an overall 1-year survival rate of 92% in patients with documented life-threatening ventricular tachyarrhythmias [26]. Three randomized, controlled trials have demonstrated the ICD to be superior to antiarrhythmic medications in the secondary prevention of SCD [27–29]. Recent primary prevention studies have also demonstrated improved survival of high-risk patients with ischemic cardiomyopathy who have had ICDs implanted as compared to conventional drug therapy [8–10, 24].

Implantable Cardioverter Defibrillators for Secondary Prevention of Sudden Cardiac Death

Following resuscitation from ventricular fibrillation (VF) or pulseless VT, ICD implantation is a proven strategy for the prevention of recurrent SCD. Three prospective, randomized, controlled trials, the Antiarrhythmics Versus Implantable Defibrillators (AVID) study, the Canadian Implantable Defibrillator Study (CIDS), and the Cardiac Arrest Study Hamburg (CASH), support this strategy [27–29].

The Canadian Implantable Defibrillator Study studied ICD therapy versus amiodarone while CASH studied ICD therapy versus a variety of antiarrhythmic medications in patients with resuscitated SCD. Both trials found nonsignificant reductions in mortality with ICD implantation. CIDS showed a relative risk (RR) reduction of 19.7% [$p = 0.14$] and CASH showed a RR reduction of 23% in mortality [$p = 0.08$].

A significant mortality benefit of ICD therapy was shown in the largest of the three studies, the AVID study. In this study, over 1,000 patients with ischemic cardiomyopathy and an EF $\leq$ 40% who were resuscitated from VF or from symptomatic, sustained VT were randomized to antiarrhythmic medications (>90% amiodarone) or ICD implantation. The trial was stopped early because the ICD showed a significant survival benefit with an 11.3% absolute and 31.5% RR reduction for all-cause mortality over 3 years. Persistent benefit with the ICD was seen even after adjustment for age, beta blocker use, and baseline EF.

A review of these three trials concluded that, compared to antiarrhythmic therapy, ICD implantation for secondary prevention results in significant reductions in all-cause mortality (RR 0.76) and SCD (RR 0.50) [30]. A meta-analysis of secondary prevention trials found an absolute reduction in all-cause mortality of 7% and a significant 25% reduction in mortality with ICD therapy compared to amiodarone that was entirely due to a 50% reduction in SCD [31]. The number needed to treat to prevent one death was 15 patients.

Evidence for Implantable Cardioverter Defibrillators for Primary Prevention of Sudden Cardiac Death

Since survival rates for out-of-hospital cardiac arrest are quite low, ranging from 2 to 25% in the United States [32], secondary prevention strategies only address a small minority of ischemic cardiomyopathy patients at risk for SCD. A more substantial reduction in SCD will result from primary prevention of SCD with ICD implantation. Evidence for this strategy comes from several recent trials. The findings of primary prevention trials for SCD in ischemic cardiomyopathy are summarized in Table 3.1.

The Multicenter Automatic Defibrillator Implantation Trial (MADIT) randomized 196 patients with ischemic cardiomyopathy, EF $\leq$ 35%, a documented episode of nonsustained VT (NSVT), and inducible VT on electrophysiology study (EPS) to ICD versus conventional medical therapy [9]. After a mean follow-up of 27 months, the RR reduction for all-cause mortality in the ICD arm was 59% [$p = 0.009$].

The Multicenter Unsustained Tachycardia Trial (MUSTT) studied a similar population of patients, with left ventricular EF $\leq$ 40% [8]. MUSTT randomized 704 patients to conventional therapy or EPS-guided therapy, consisting of antiarrhythmic medication or ICD implantation if at least one antiarrhythmic medication was ineffective at suppressing inducible VT on EPS. At 5 years, patients receiving EPS-guided therapy had significant reduction in arrhythmic death and an almost significant reduction in total mortality. Reduction in both end points in the EPS-guided group was entirely attributable to the ICD, as there was no difference in outcome between patients receiving no additional therapy and those treated with antiarrhythmic medication (Fig. 3.3).

Table 3.1 Summary of ICD primary prevention trials in ischemic cardiomyopathy

Study	Design	No. of Pts	Mean follow up (months)	Results	P value
MADIT (NEJM 1996)	ICD vs pharmacotherapy (74% amiodarone) in preventing sudden death in patients with old MI and NSVT, EF $\leq 35\%$	196	27	All cause mortality reduction by 54% in ICD arm	$= 0.009$
MUSTT (NEJM 1999)	EP guided therapy (antiarrhythmic drugs and ICD) vs no therapy in patients with CAD, EF $\leq 40\%$, asymptomatic NSVT and inducible VT with EP study	704	39	All cause mortality reduced by 55% in ICD arm (compared to control), arrhythmic death reduced by 73%	<0.001 <0.001
MADIT II (NEJM 2002)	ICD vs conventional therapy in prevention of mortality in patients with CAD, an old MI and EF $\leq 30\%$	1,232	20 Stopped early by DSMB	All cause mortality reduction by 31% in ICD arm	$= 0.016$
COMPANION (NEJM 2004)	Optimal pharmacological therapy (OPT) vs chronic resynchronization therapy (CRT) vs CRT + an implantable defibrillator (CRT-D) in patients with CHF NYHA III–IV, EF $\leq 35\%$, QRS > 120 ms	1,520	15 Stopped early by DSMB	Death or hospitalization for CHF reduced by 34% in CRT, 40% in CRT-D	<0.002 <0.001
SCD-HeFT (NEJM 2005)	Conventional therapy vs Amiodarone vs ICD in patients with CHF NYHA III–IV, EF $\leq 35\%$	2,521	45.5	All cause mortality reduction by 23% in ICD arm	$= 0.007$
CABG PATCH (NEJM 1997)	ICD vs no ICD in patients with CAD, EF $\leq 35\%$, abnormal SAECG undergoing CABG	900	32	No difference in all cause mortality	$= 0.64$
DINAMIT (NEJM 2004)	ICD vs no ICD in patients with recent MI (6–40 days), EF $\leq 35\%$ and impaired cardiac autonomic function	674	30	No difference in all cause mortality reduction	$= 0.66$

CABG PATCH = Coronary Artery Bypass Graft (CABG) Patch Trial.
CAD = Coronary Artery Disease.
CHF = Congestive Heart Failure.
COMPANION = Comparison of Medical therapy, Resynchronization, and Defibrillation therapies in Heart failure.
CRT = Cardiac Resynchronization Therapy.
DEFINITE = Defibrillators in Non-Ischemic Cardiomyopathy Treatment Evaluation Investigators.
DINAMIT = Defibrillator in Acute Myocardial Infarction Trial.
DSMB = Data Safety Monitoring Board.
EF = Ejection Fraction.
ICD = Implantable Cardiac Defibrillator.
MADIT = Multicenter Automatic Defibrillator Implantation Trial.
MI = Myocardial Infarction.
MUSTT = Multicenter UnSustained Tachycardia Trial.
NEJM = New England Journal of Medicine.
NSVT = Non Sustained Ventricular Tachycardia.
NYHA = New York Heart Association.
PVC = Premature Ventricular Contraction.
SAECG = Signal Averaged Electrocardiogram.
SCD-HeFT = Sudden Cardiac Death in Heart Failure Trial.

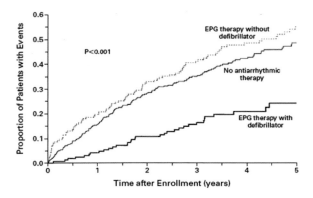

Fig. 3.3 Overall mortality rates for those receiving no anti-arrhythmic medication, EPS-guided therapy without ICD (antiarrhythmic medication), and those receiving ICD in the MUSTT study

Because the above trials showed a >50% relative reduction in total mortality with ICD therapy, MADIT II used broader entry criteria for primary prevention of SCD, removing the criteria for NSVT and EPS; 1,232 patients with a history of MI > 30 days prior and an EF ≤ 30% were randomized to conventional therapy or ICD implantation [10]. "Conventional therapy" was comparable in both arms and included a high rate of use of beta block-ers, angiotensin-converting enzyme inhibitors, and statins (over two thirds for all medications in both arms). The trial was stopped early at 20 months because the relative reduction in total mortality

was 31% in the ICD arm (Fig. 3.4). The survival benefit was entirely due to a reduction in SCD.

Survival curves in MADIT II did not separate until 9 months after enrollment, raising the question of when an ICD should be implanted after MI or revascularization. Two notable negative primary prevention trials may answer this question. The Coronary Artery Bypass Graft Patch (CABG-Patch) Trial evaluated whether primary prevention with ICD at the time of surgical revascularization in patients with EF ≤ 35% and a positive SAECG would reduce total mortality [33]. At 32 months follow-up, no difference was found, suggesting that there is no additional benefit to ICD therapy at the time of revascularization.

The Defibrillator in Acute Myocardial Infarction Trial (DINAMIT) enrolled nearly 700 patients with recent MI, ranging from 6 to 40 days (median 7 days), EF < 36%, and reduced heart rate variability but without NYHA class IV symptoms, sustained VT within 48 h of MI, or surgical or percutaneous 3-vessel revascularization [34]. Patients were randomized to ICD therapy versus conventional therapy and at 1 year, there was no difference in total mortality with more arrhythmic deaths in the control arm and more nonarrhythmic deaths in the ICD arm. Thus, there appears to be no benefit to ICD therapy in the immediate post-MI period. An interpretation of the negative result of both of these trials is that significant recovery of LV function may have occurred in the

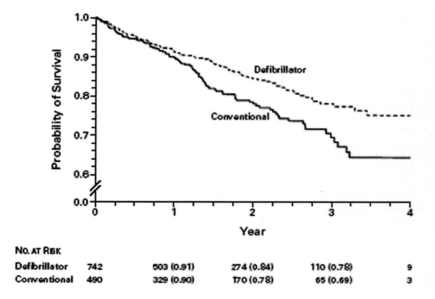

Fig. 3.4 Survival rates for patients receiving conventional therapy versus those receiving ICD therapy in MADIT II

NO. AT RISK					
Defibrillator	742	503 (0.91)	274 (0.84)	110 (0.78)	9
Conventional	490	329 (0.90)	170 (0.78)	65 (0.69)	3

studied population in the immediate period following acute MI or surgical revascularization. However, in direct contrast to DINAMIT, a recent substudy of VALIANT (Valsartan in Acute Myocardial Infarction Trial) found that the risk of SCD is highest in the first 30 days after MI among patients with LV dysfunction, heart failure, or both [35]. Therefore, the timing of ICD implantation after MI in the setting of LV dysfunction may still be open to debate.

The results of MADIT II were met with some skepticism, but later confirmed by the recent Sudden Cardiac Death in Heart Failure Trial (SCD-HeFT) [24]. This study evaluated the benefit of ICD therapy versus amiodarone or placebo as primary prevention in over 2,500 patients with stable NYHA class II or III heart failure and EF $\leq$ 35%, without the requirement for NSVT or EPS. Patients with both ischemic and nonischemic etiologies for cardiomyopathy were included. Over a follow-up of 4 years, there was no benefit of amiodarone over placebo for overall mortality, but ICD therapy resulted in a significant 23% reduction in overall mortality [$p = 0.007$] (Fig. 3.5). The benefit of ICD therapy was comparable for ischemic and nonischemic cardiomyopathy.

The DEFINITE (The Defibrillators in Non-Ischemic Cardiomyopathy Treatment Evaluation) trial focused on ICD use only in patients with nonischemic cardiomyopathy [36]. This trial randomized 458 patients with documented nonischemic cardiomyopathy, LVEF < 36%, New York Heart Association (NYHA) Class I–III, and arrhythmia markers (premature ventricular complexes or non-sustained VT on Holter monitoring) to either standard medical therapy or standard medical therapy plus ICD. The primary endpoint of the study was death from any cause; the secondary endpoint was sudden death from arrhythmia. After 1 year follow-up, the death rate from any cause was 2.6% in the ICD group versus 6.2% in the standard medical therapy group, and at the end of 2 years, the rates were 7.9 and 14.1%, respectively. This difference in mortality was entirely due to reduction in arrhythmia related mortality.

Summary of Evidence and Current Guidelines

A meta-analysis performed before SCD-HeFT synthesized the evidence for ICD implantation in primary and secondary prevention [30]. The RR for SCD with ICDs in primary prevention was 37%

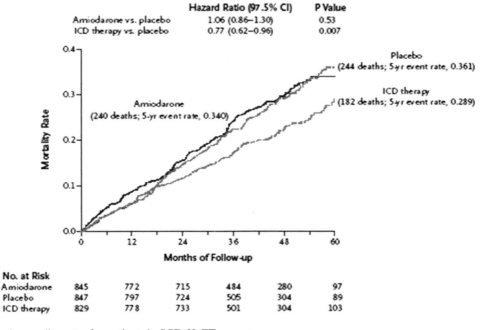

Fig. 3.5 Total mortality rates for patients in SCD-HeFT

and that for secondary prevention 50%. ICDs as primary prevention were also highly efficacious in reducing total mortality (RR 0.72). Of note, greater benefit was seen in studies enrolling patients at higher risk, as in MUSTT or MADIT, as compared to those at lower risk, as in MADIT II.

As a result of the weight of evidence for ICD therapy in prevention of SCD in patients with ischemic cardiomyopathy, the American College of Cardiology, American Heart Association, and the North American Society for Pacing and Electrophysiology (now Heart Rhythm Society) revised guidelines for ICD implantation in October 2002 [37].Over the years, guidelines have evolved with publications of additional trials. The most recent guidelines, published in May, 2008, have combined and extended upon the criteria of individual trials [38]. These guidelines, as applicable to heart failure patients, are summarized in Table 3.2. Of significance was the upgrade of recommendation for prophylactic ICD implantation in patients with EF $\leq$ 30%, $\geq$1 month after MI, and $\geq$3 months after revascularization, NYHA class I from Class IIA to Class I. Also, ICD therapy in patients with LVEF less than 35% due to prior MI who are at least 40 days post-MI and are in NYHA functional Class II or III remained a Class I indication, although the EF cutoff (<35%) was lower compared to the 2006 guidelines.

The Centers for Medicare and Medicaid Services reimbursement criteria for ICDs (http://www.cms.hhs. gov/mcd/viewimplementation.asp?id = 148) include patients with either ischemic or nonischemic cardiomyopathy with EF $\leq$ 35%, and NYHA class II or III heart failure, removing the controversial criteria from 2003 which restricted ICDs to patients with ischemic cardiomyopathy, EF $\leq$ 30%, and QRS > 120 ms. Patients with ischemic cardiomyopathy must not have undergone revascularization within 3 months nor had MI within 40 days. All patients who receive ICDs for primary prevention are included in a national registry in the hopes of further defining risks, benefits, and indications.

Prevention of Harm in Patients with Implantable Cardioverter Defibrillators

Modern transvenous ICD implantation procedures are associated with very low complication (bleeding, infection, pneumothorax, failed implantation) rates [39, 40]. Following implantation, complications include failed or inappropriate shocks, and lead fractures, infection, or dislodgment. In addition, although potentially lifesaving, ICD shocks are not only physically painful, they result in a significant amount of psychological stress and burden for patients with ICDs. In fact, panic disorders and agoraphobia are well-recognized side effects of ICD shocks [41]. Therefore, strategies to reduce ICD shocks would greatly benefit quality of life for patients with ICDs.

One very effective strategy is antitachycardia pacing (ATP), a capability which is incorporated in most ICDs. ATP painlessly terminates sustained

Table 3.2 ACC/AHA/HRS updated guidelines for implantation of ICDs, May 2008

Indication for ICD	Level of evidence	Strength of recommendation
Survivors of cardiac arrest due to VF or hemodynamically unstable sustained VT after evaluation to define the cause of the event and to exclude any completely reversible causes	A	Class I
Patients with LVEF less than 35% due to prior MI who are at least 40 days post-MI and are in NYHA functional Class II or III	A	Class I
Patients with nonischemic cardiomyopathy who have an LVEF less than or equal to 35% and who are in NYHA functional Class II or II	B	Class I
Patients with LV dysfunction due to prior MI who are at least 40 days post-MI, have an LVEF less than 30%, and are in NYHA functional Class I	A	Class I
Patients with nonsustained VT due to prior MI, LVEF less than 40%, and inducible VF or sustained VT at electrophysiological study	B	Class I
Patients with structural heart disease and spontaneous sustained VT, whether hemodynamically stable or unstable	B	Class I

VT with overdrive pacing, thus reducing the number of ICD shocks and improving patient comfort. ATP successfully terminates between 77 and 91% of fast VT with a very low rate (4%) of acceleration and syncope [42, 43].

Another issue is the risk of worsening heart failure with ICDs. The MADIT II study showed a slightly higher rate of hospitalization for heart failure in the ICD arm that was not seen in the control arm (20 versus 15%). A MADIT II analysis showed that patients who received dual chamber devices (and thus had ventricular pacing) had higher risk of heart failure hospitalization without difference in mortality. This observation was confirmed in the Dual Chamber and VVI Implantable Defibrillator (DAVID) trial, in which unnecessary right ventricular pacing (and thus pacing-induced ventricular dyssynchrony) resulted in higher rates of heart failure hospitalizations [44]. This interpretation is in accord with the evidence for benefit of biventricular pacing (resynchronization therapy) in heart failure and the results from SCD-HeFT, which did not show an increase in heart failure hospitalizations because ICDs were programmed for back-up pacing only below heart rates of 34 beats per minute.

Implementation and Cost of Implantable Cardioverter Defibrillators

Implantable cardioverter defibrillator implantations have increased dramatically over the last decade [45], with a 24% worldwide annual increase in ICD implantations between 1998 and 2002 [1]. There was an increase in the number of Medicare beneficiaries eligible for ICDs by two- to threefold, to more than 500,000, based on the most recent reimbursement criteria [46].

Implantable cardioverter defibrillator implantation is expensive, with an estimated cost of $30,000–$50,000 per implant, not including the cost of follow-up. However, economic analysis of ICD studies has shown that ICD implantation compares favorably with such commonly accepted therapies as dialysis for end-stage renal failure [47]. It is estimated that the cost effectiveness ratio for ICDs is $27,000 per life year saved, comparable to those for other well-

accepted cardiac interventions as CABG ($18,200), cardiac transplant ($44,300), and percutaneous coronary angioplasty for 1-vessel disease in patients with mild angina ($91,500) [1].

As demand and supply increase, along with technological advances, it is anticipated that ICD costs will gradually decrease, thus further improving cost effectiveness. Because the majority of patients receiving ICDs for primary prevention will never trigger a therapy (shock), cost effectiveness can be further maximized by identifying those at highest risk for SCD and avoiding ICD implantation in those unlikely to suffer SCD. To this end, investigators have demonstrated the utility of additional risk stratification with microvolt T-wave alternans in predicting which MADIT II patients are likely to benefit from ICD therapy, although this has not yet been prospectively validated [15], and others are examining the role of genetics in predicting SCD.

References

1. Seidl K, Senges J. Worldwide utilization of implantable cardioverter/defibrillators now and in the future. *Card Electrophysiol Rev*.Jan 2003;7(1):5–13.
2. State-specific mortality from sudden cardiac death—United States, 1999. *MMWR Morb Mortal Wkly Rep*.Feb 15 2002;51(6):123–126.
3. Kannel WB, Thomas HE, Jr. Sudden coronary death: the Framingham study. *Ann N Y Acad Sci*.1982;382:3–21.
4. Zheng ZJ, Croft JB, Giles WH, et al. Sudden cardiac death in the United States, 1989 to 1998. *Circulation*. Oct 30 2001;104(18):2158–2163.
5. Huikuri HV, Castellanos A, Myerburg RJ. Sudden death due to cardiac arrhythmias. *N Engl J Med*. Nov 15 2001;345(20):1473–1482.
6. Zipes DP, Wellens HJ. Sudden cardiac death. *Circulation*. Nov 24 1998;98(21):2334–2351.
7. Myerburg RJ, Kessler KM, Castellanos A. Sudden cardiac death. Structure, function, and time-dependence of risk. *Circulation*. Jan 1992;85(1 Suppl):I2–I10.
8. Buxton AE, Lee KL, Fisher JD, et al. A randomized study of the prevention of sudden death in patients with coronary artery disease. Multicenter unsustained tachycardia trial investigators. *N Engl J Med*. Dec 16 1999;341(25):1882–1890.
9. Moss AJ, Hall WJ, Cannom DS, et al. Improved survival with an implanted defibrillator in patients with coronary disease at high risk for ventricular arrhythmia. Multicenter automatic defibrillator implantation trial investigators. *N Engl J Med*.Dec 26 1996;335(26):1933–1940.
10. Moss AJ, Zareba W, Hall WJ, et al. Prophylactic implantation of a defibrillator in patients with myocardial

infarction and reduced ejection fraction. *N Engl J Med.* Mar 21 2002;346(12):877–883.

11. MERIT-HF Study Group. Effect of metoprolol CR/XL in chronic heart failure: Metoprolol CR/XL randomised intervention trial in congestive heart failure (MERIT-HF). *Lancet.* Jun 12 1999;353(9169):2001–2007.

12. Friedlander Y, Siscovick DS, Weinmann S, et al. Family history as a risk factor for primary cardiac arrest. *Circulation.* Jan 20 1998;97(2):155–160.

13. Jouven X, Desnos M, Guerot C, et al. Predicting sudden death in the population: the Paris prospective study I. *Circulation.* Apr 20 1999;99(15):1978–1983.

14. Huikuri HV, Makikallio TH, Raatikainen MJ, et al. Prediction of sudden cardiac death: appraisal of the studies and methods assessing the risk of sudden arrhythmic death. *Circulation.* Jul 8 2003;108(1):110–115.

15. Bloomfield DM, Steinman RC, Namerow PB, et al. Microvolt T-wave alternans distinguishes between patients likely and patients not likely to benefit from implanted cardiac defibrillator therapy: a solution to the multicenter automatic defibrillator implantation trial (MADIT) II conundrum. *Circulation.* Oct 5 2004;110(14):1885–1889.

16. Klingenheben T, Hohnloser SH. Clinical value of T-wave alternans assessment. *Card Electrophysiol Rev.* Sep 2002;6(3):323–328.

17. Buxton AE, Lee KL, DiCarlo L, et al. Electrophysiologic testing to identify patients with coronary artery disease who are at risk for sudden death. Multicenter unsustained tachycardia trial investigators. *N Engl J Med.* Jun 29 2000;342(26):1937–1945.

18. Wood M, Stambler B, Ellenbogen K. Recent insights in programmed electrical stimulation for the management of sustained ventricular arrhythmias. *Curr Opin Cardiol.* Jan 1994;9(1):3–11.

19. Andresen D, Steinbeck G, Bruggemann T, et al. Risk stratification following myocardial infarction in the thrombolytic era: a two-step strategy using noninvasive and invasive methods. *J Am Coll Cardiol.* Jan 1999;33(1):131–138.

20. Effect of the antiarrhythmic agent moricizine on survival after myocardial infarction. The cardiac arrhythmia suppression trial II investigators. *N Engl J Med.* Jul 23 1992;327(4):227–233.

21. The cardiac arrhythmia suppression trial. *N Engl J Med.* Dec 21 1989;321(25):1754–1756.

22. Cairns JA, Connolly SJ, Roberts R, et al. Randomised trial of outcome after myocardial infarction in patients with frequent or repetitive ventricular premature depolarisations: CAMIAT. Canadian Amiodarone myocardial infarction arrhythmia trial investigators. *Lancet.* Mar 8 1997;349(9053):675–682.

23. Julian DG, Camm AJ, Frangin G, et al. Randomised trial of effect of amiodarone on mortality in patients with left-ventricular dysfunction after recent myocardial infarction: EMIAT. European myocardial infarct amiodarone trial investigators. *Lancet.* Mar 8 1997;349(9053):667–674.

24. Bardy GH, Lee KL, Mark DB, et al. Amiodarone or an implantable cardioverter-defibrillator for congestive heart failure. *N Engl J Med.* Jan 20 2005;352(3):225–237.

25. Yusuf S, Peto R, Lewis J, et al. Beta blockade during and after myocardial infarction: an overview of the randomized trials. *Prog Cardiovasc Dis.* Mar–Apr 1985;27(5):335–371.

26. Winkle RA, Mead RH, Ruder MA, et al. Long-term outcome with the automatic implantable cardioverter-defibrillator. *J Am Coll Cardiol.* May 1989;13(6):1353–1361.

27. A comparison of antiarrhythmic-drug therapy with implantable defibrillators in patients resuscitated from near-fatal ventricular arrhythmias. The antiarrhythmics versus implantable defibrillators (AVID) investigators. *N Engl J Med.* Nov 27 1997;337(22):1576–1583.

28. Kuck KH, Cappato R, Siebels J, et al. Randomized comparison of antiarrhythmic drug therapy with implantable defibrillators in patients resuscitated from cardiac arrest: the Cardiac Arrest Study Hamburg (CASH). *Circulation.* Aug 15 2000;102(7):748–754.

29. Connolly SJ, Gent M, Roberts RS, et al. Canadian implantable defibrillator study (CIDS): a randomized trial of the implantable cardioverter defibrillator against amiodarone. *Circulation.* Mar 21 2000;101(11):1297–1302.

30. Ezekowitz JA, Armstrong PW, McAlister FA. Implantable cardioverter defibrillators in primary and secondary prevention: a systematic review of randomized, controlled trials. *Ann Intern Med.* Mar 18 2003;138(6):445–452.

31. Lee DS, Green LD, Liu PP, et al. Effectiveness of implantable defibrillators for preventing arrhythmic events and death: a meta-analysis. *J Am Coll Cardiol.* May 7 2003;41(9):1573–1582.

32. Eisenberg MS, Horwood BT, Cummins RO, et al. Cardiac arrest and resuscitation: a tale of 29 cities. *Ann Emerg Med.* Feb 1990;19(2):179–186.

33. Bigger JT, Jr. Prophylactic use of implanted cardiac defibrillators in patients at high risk for ventricular arrhythmias after coronary-artery bypass graft surgery. Coronary artery bypass graft (CABG) patch trial investigators. *N Engl J Med.* Nov 27 1997;337(22):1569–1575.

34. Hohnloser SH, Kuck KH, Dorian P, et al. Prophylactic use of an implantable cardioverter-defibrillator after acute myocardial infarction. *N Engl J Med.* Dec 9 2004;351(24):2481–2488.

35. Solomon SD, Zelenkofske S, McMurray JJ, et al. Sudden death in patients with myocardial infarction and left ventricular dysfunction, heart failure, or both. *N Engl J Med.* Jun 23 2005;352(25):2581–2588.

36. Kadish A, Dyer A, Daubert JP, et al., for the Defibrillators in Non-Ischemic Cardiomyopathy Treatment Evaluation (DEFINITE) Investigators. Prophylactic defibrillator implantation in patients with nonischemic dilated cardiomyopathy. *N Engl J Med.* 2004;350:2151–2158.

37. Gregoratos G, Abrams J, Epstein AE, et al. ACC/AHA/NASPE 2002 guideline update for implantation of cardiac pacemakers and antiarrhythmia devices: summary article: a report of the American College of Cardiology/American Heart Association Task Force on Practice Guidelines (ACC/AHA/NASPE Committee to Update the 1998 Pacemaker Guidelines). *Circulation.* Oct 15 2002;106(16):2145–2161.

38. Andrew EE, John PD, Kenneth AE, et al. ACC/AHA/HRS 2008 guidelines for device-based therapy of cardiac rhythm abnormalities. *J Am Coll Cardiol*. 2008;51:1–62.

39. Anvari A, Stix G, Grabenwoger M, et al. Comparison of three cardioverter defibrillator implantation techniques: initial results with transvenous pectoral implantation. *Pacing Clin Electrophysiol*. Jul 1996;19(7):1061–1069.

40. Cardinal DS, Connelly DT, Steinhaus DM, et al. Cost savings with nonthoracotomy implantable cardioverter-defibrillators. *Am J Cardiol*. Dec 1 1996;78(11):1255–1259.

41. Godemann F, Butter C, Lampe F, et al. Panic disorders and agoraphobia: side effects of treatment with an implantable cardioverter/defibrillator. *Clin Cardiol*. Jun 2004;27(6):321–326.

42. Fromer M, Brachmann J, Block M, et al. Efficacy of automatic multimodal device therapy for ventricular tachyarrhythmias as delivered by a new implantable pacing cardioverter-defibrillator. Results of a European multicenter study of 102 implants. *Circulation*. Aug 1992;86(2):363–374.

43. Wathen MS, Sweeney MO, DeGroot PJ, et al. Shock reduction using antitachycardia pacing for spontaneous rapid ventricular tachycardia in patients with coronary artery disease. *Circulation*. Aug 14 2001;104(7):796–801.

44. Schron EB, Exner DV, Yao Q, et al. Quality of life in the antiarrhythmics versus implantable defibrillators trial: impact of therapy and influence of adverse symptoms and defibrillator shocks. *Circulation*. Feb 5 2002;105(5):589–594.

45. Higgins SL. Impact of the multicenter automatic defibrillator implantation trial on implantable cardioverter defibrillator indication trends. *Am J Cardiol*. Mar 11 1999;83(5B):79D–82D.

46. McClellan MB, Tunis SR. Medicare coverage of ICDs. *N Engl J Med*. Jan 20 2005;352(3):222–224.

47. Morgan JM. Cost-effectiveness of implantable cardioverter defibrillator therapy. *J Cardiovasc Electrophysiol*. Jan 2002;13(1 Suppl):S114–S117.

Chapter 4
Pacemaker Therapy for Advanced Ischemic Heart Disease

Explanation of Cardiac Resynchronization Therapy and Its Role in Treating AIHD

John P. Boehmer

Conduction System Disease in Ischemic Heart Disease

Conduction system abnormalities are common in chronic heart failure, occurring in 15–30% of the population with low left ventricular ejection fraction (LVEF) [1–3]. The prevalence in ischemic heart disease is roughly similar to that seen in other forms of dilated cardiomyopathy. Conduction system disease can occur both at the time of an acute myocardial infarction as well as slowly progressing in chronic ischemic heart disease. Intraventricular conduction delays are associated with a poor prognosis in heart failure, with up to a 70% increase in the risk of death, and are also more prevalent in patients with advanced symptoms [2, 4]. In ischemic heart disease, all components of the conduction system are at risk of ischemic injury, from the sinoatrial node to the His-Pukinje system. These conduction system abnormalities have the potential to impair cardiac function by a number of mechanisms. Since conduction abnormalities impair cardiac function, it is logical that pacing therapies to correct or improve these conduction abnormalities may improve cardiac function.

Anatomy and Physiology of the Normal Conduction System

The sinus node initiates a heartbeat and is located laterally in the epicardial groove of the sulcus terminalis, near the junction of the superior vena cava and right atrium. The sinus node is comprised of "nests" of principal pacemaker cells, which spontaneously depolarize and are situated within a fibrous tissue matrix. Rather than being a discreet point of impulse initiation, the sinus node is in reality a "region" [5]. In addition to the nest of principal pacemaker cells, other nests contain cells with slower intrinsic depolarization rates and serve as backup pacemakers in response to changing physiological and pathological conditions. Therefore, the principal pacemaker site shifts within the sinus nodal region, which may result in subtle changes in P-wave morphology [6]. The blood supply to this region predominantly comes from the sinus nodal artery, which is a branch of the right coronary artery in 65% of patients, although there is variability of coronary anatomy and blood supply to the region [7].

The AV node lies directly above the insertion of the septal leaflet of the tricuspid valve and anterior to the ostium of the coronary sinus. It is part of the AV junction area, which is divided into three regions. The transitional cells, or nodal approaches, connect the atrial myocardium to the compact portion of the AV node. The slowest conduction time occurs within the AV node [8]. At its distal end, the compact portion of the AV node enters the central fibrous body, becoming the penetrating portion, or His-bundle [9].

J.P. Boehmer (✉)
Division of Cardiology, The Heart and Vascular Institute, The Penn State Hershey Medical Center, The Pennsylvania State University College of Medicine, Hershey, PA 17033, USA
e-mail: jboehmer@psu.edu

R. Delgado, H.S. Arora (eds.), *Interventional Treatment of Advanced Ischemic Heart Disease*,
DOI 10.1007/978-1-84800-395-8_4, © Springer-Verlag London Limited 2009

The blood supply to the AV node is via the AV nodal artery, a branch of the right coronary artery in 90% of hearts, with the remaining 10% arising from the circumflex artery [10]. The main His bundle is typically supplied by the AV nodal artery with a minor contribution from septal perforators, but the bundle branches have a blood supply that is more dependent on septal perforators.

After leaving the AV node, the bundle of His divides into the right and left bundle branches near the juncture of the membranous and muscular interventricular septa. The right bundle travels near the endocardium in its upper third and lower third, being deeper in the myocardium through the middle third. The main blood supply is from septal perforators from the LAD. It begins to ramify as it approaches the right anterior papillary muscle with fascicles going first to the septum and then to the right ventricular free wall. The main left bundle branch penetrates the membranous interventricular septum under the aortic ring, and then divides into two or three fairly discrete branches [8, 11–13]. The left bundle obtains the majority of its blood supply from the LAD before dividing. The anterior fascicle crosses the left ventricular (LV) outflow tract and supplies the anterolateral wall of the left ventricle. The anterior fascicle is supplied by septal perforators from the LAD and in about 50% of patients from the AV nodal artery. The posterior fascicle extends out inferiorly and posteriorly. Septal perforators from the LAD supply the proximal portion of the posterior fascicle, but the distal portion receives blood supply from both anterior and posterior septal perforators. In about 65% of hearts, there is a separate fascicle to the interventricular septum.

Conduction Disturbances During Acute Myocardial Infarction

Although much of the data regarding the frequency of conduction abnormalities during acute myocardial infarction were derived from studies prior to the era of rapid reperfusion [14–17], data from more recent trials suggest that the incidence of intraventricular conduction defects has changed very little,

occurring in 10–20% of patients [18, 19]. In contrast, the incidence of complete heart block appears to have decreased from 5 to 9% in the prethrombolytic era to 4–5% more recently. A report of patients in the Thrombolysis and Angioplasty in Myocardial Infarction (TIMI) 9 and Global Utilization of Streptokinase and t-PA for Occluded Arteries (GUSTO) 1 protocols revealed an overall incidence of bundle branch block of 23.6% with 5.3% of patients having persistent bundle branch block [20]. Right bundle branch block was found in 13% of the population; left bundle branch block was found in 7%, and alternating bundle branch block was seen in 3.5%. Patients with bundle branch blocks were more likely to have left anterior descending artery infarcts (54%), lower ejection fractions, larger infarcts, and more diseased coronary arteries.

A higher mortality was seen in patients with bundle branch blocks than those without (8.7% and 3.5%, respectively; $P < 0.007$) with the highest mortality occurring in those with persistent bundle branch block (mortality 19.4%) [20]. The increase in risk of death is similar to that seen in the Swedish Register of Information and Knowledge about Swedish Heart Intensive care Admissions, where data from 88,026 cases of myocardial infarction were included [21]. This was an inclusive database from 72 hospitals in Sweden over a 6-year time period. The 1-year mortality for patients with LBBB was 42% and 22% for those without LBBB. However, the presence of LBBB was correlated with a number of other poor prognostic factors including age, concomitant diseases, and LVEF. After controlling for these factors, the relative risk of death for those with LBBB was 1.19, 95% confidence interval 1.14–1.24, $P < 0.001$. Therefore, the majority of the increase in mortality could be assigned to associated risk factors, but not the entire increased risk.

Sinus Node Dysfunction in Heart Failure

Chronic heart failure is associated with intrinsic sinus node dysfunction that can be demonstrated on careful electrophysiologic studies [22, 23]. Patients with chronic heart failure have longer intrinsic sinus cycle length, or slower heart rates when isolated from autonomic influence. There is prolongation of the corrected sinus node recovery time. There are further anatomical and functional changes that include more caudal location of sinus activity, prolonged sinoatrail conduction time, and greater number and duration of fractionated electrograms along the crista terminalis. The intrinsic sinus node dysfunction is exacerbated by many of the drugs necessary to treat heart failure with advanced ischemic heart disease, including beta blockers, digoxin, and some antiarrhythmic drugs. Subsequent atrial depolarization is also associated with delayed conduction that can be detected in the low right atrium and along the coronary sinus. This can create timing delays between atrial and ventricular contraction in the absence of AV nodal or His-Purkinje disease.

Sinus bradycardia can be found patients with chronic heart failure, particularly when treated aggressively with beta blockers and antiarrhythmic drugs such as amiodarone [24]. Most patients will not have syncope or near-syncope as a symptom. However, fatigue and exercise intolerance are common symptoms in patients with heart failure, and the relationship of these symptoms to mild resting bradycardia is unclear. A 12-lead ECG is commonly obtained, but rarely provides definitive information about sinus node function. A 24 h ambulatory ECG monitor can provide information about the occurrence of sinus pauses and association with symptoms recording in the accompanying diary. However, several studies have demonstrated the futility of treating asymptomatic pauses, as most pauses, ranging from 2 to 15 s, are asymptomatic and pacing does not benefit those without associated symptoms [25, 26]. Exercise testing can be useful to identify patients with chronotropic incompetence, and this is likely important in the setting of compensated chronic heart failure where many patients may have resting bradycardia, but reasonably preserved exercise heart rate response. In this situation, atrial pacing is likely to be of little benefit.

The symptom of syncope in a patient with ischemic heart disease and heart failure should initially prompt concern about ventricular dysrhythmias. Based on the results of recent clinical trials of sudden death prevention in heart failure [27, 28], most patients with low ejection fraction and advanced ischemic heart disease will likely be treated with an implantable cardioverter-defibrillator. However, for patients with higher ejection fractions, other electrical causes of syncope must be considered as well, since such patients are at risk for disease throughout the conduction system. In the elderly patients with paroxysmal atrial fibrillation, syncope is classically associated with a long sinus pause at the spontaneous termination of the tachycardia. Electrophysiologic studies can also be used to assess sinus node function, but this is usually reserved for patients who are symptomatic, and noninvasive study fails to demonstrate an etiology to their symptoms.

Treatment

Ideally, if symptomatic sinus node dysfunction occurs in the presence of drugs known to impair sinus node function, the first treatment is to discontinue the offending drug [29]. However, this is typically not feasible in patients with heart failure who are dependent on several medications to improve long-term outcomes, or may need antiarrhythmic drug therapy for symptomatic arrhythmias. Accordingly, the treatment usually becomes a question of whether to apply pacing to increase heart rate. This is further complicated by the appropriate pacemaker prescription once the decision to pace has been made.

Many experienced clinicians feel that the benefit from beta blocker therapy is sufficient to justify permanent pacing while maintaining beta blocker therapy [24, 30]. It should be noted that patients with very low resting heart rates or symptomatic bradycardia were excluded from beta blocker mortality trials and the utilization of permanent pacing during these trials was very low [31–34]. Accordingly, there are few data to support the strategy of utilizing permanent pacing for atrial rate support. Additionally, care must be taken in advanced ischemic heart disease to avoid the induction of ischemia with higher heart rates, since heart rate is a primary determinant of myocardial oxygen consumption.

There is only one randomized controlled clinical trial of pacing therapy to increase heart rates in patients with chronic heart failure and that is the

Dual Chamber and VVI Implantable Defibrillator (DAVID) trial [30]. The rationale of this trial was that the sinus node dysfunction inherent in chronic heart failure and exacerbated by pharmacologic therapy leads to a decrease in the doses of therapeutic medication. The hypothesis was that dual chamber pacing would permit optimal pharmacologic therapy and improve hemodynamics, thereby reducing the morbidity associated with heart failure. In this study, patients who had chronic heart failure and a standard indication for ICD implantation, but without an indication for anti-bradycardia pacing, were implanted with a dual chamber ICD, then randomized to one of two pacing modes, DDDR at 70 bpm (250 patients) or VVI at 40 bpm (256 patients). The patients randomized to DDDR pacing had worse outcomes, including an increase in the primary endpoint of combined death or heart failure hospitalization (16.1% in VVI group versus 26.7% in the DDDR group, relative hazard 1.61; CI 1.06–2.44; see Fig. 4.1), a trend to an increase in all-cause death (6.5% in VVI group versus 10.1% in DDDR group, relative hazard 1.61, 95% CI 0.84–3.09), and hospitalization for worsening heart failure (13.3% for the VVI group versus 22.6% for the DDDR group, relative hazard 1.54; 95% CI 0.97–2.46). In a post-hoc analysis, the adverse events were correlated with the frequency of right ventricular pacing. Although there are clear adverse effects of right ventricular pacing that will be discussed later in this chapter, the principal hypothesis of the study was that higher heart rates would improve outcomes, and this did not occur in any subgroup analysis.

The clear message from the DAVID trial was to aggressively avoid right ventricular pacing in heart failure patients, particularly in patients with narrow QRS complexes. Beyond this, we have very little data from large-scale studies to determine pacing prescription. However, several observations may provide some guiding principals. Long-term heart rate slowing improves ventricular function in animal models of systolic dysfunction [35, 36]. Additionally, slow heart rates are an energetically more favorable condition [37] and patients with chronic heart failure have been shown to be relatively energetically depleted [38, 39]. However, patients with only mild symptomatic impairment often have relatively preserved heart rate response to exercise, while those with advanced heart failure symptoms tend to have lower peak exercise heart rates [40–44]. Accordingly, one might argue to utilize the lowest resting heart rate possible while providing at least a reasonably physiologic response to exercise. While a higher peak exercise heart rate may improve functional capacity in patients with documented chronotropic incompetence, care must be taken in advanced ischemic heart disease to avoid the induction of ischemia by aggressive use of rate responsive pacing.

AV Synchrony

In the normal situation, the sinus node initiates a wave of depolarization that spreads rapidly throughout both atria. The atria contract followed shortly thereafter by contraction of the

Fig. 4.1 Event-free survival for death or hospitalization for new or worsening heart failure in the DAVID trial. Time to death or first hospitalization for new or worsening heart failure in the DAVID trial. CI indicates confidence interval. Unadjusted $P = 0.02$, $P = 0.03$ adjusted for sequential monitoring

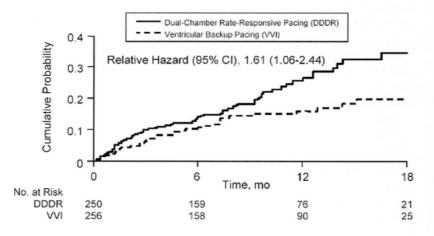

ventricles. The contraction of the atria provide filling of the ventricles beyond what occurs by passive filling [45–47]. However, if the atrial contribution to LV filling is completed too early, some of the additional preload may flow back into the atria during late diastole, which is the so-called diastolic mitral regurgitation [46–50]. Therefore, timing is important to allow the atria to maximally empty into the ventricles just prior to the initiation of systole. The additional preload provided by the atria may increase both the force of ventricular contraction and stroke volume [45, 51, 52]. The net result is an increase in cardiac output that may be as high as 25% in some patients.

Studies evaluating pacing solely for improving AV synchrony in heart failure patients reveal mixed results [45, 53–57]. The confusion in the literature may be related to a number of variables that come into play when providing AV synchronized pacing, including whether the atria are paced or used solely to trigger ventricular pacing, the heart rate provided if atrial pacing is used, the inter-atrial conduction delay, and the precise timing of ventricular stimulation to initiate systole at maximal preload provided by the atria. However, the parameter that may be most implicated is the induction of dyssynchrony within the ventricles by right ventricular pacing. Right ventricular pacing initiates a wave of depolarization and subsequent mechanical activation of the ventricles that begins on the right side of the interventricular septum and activates the LV free wall late [58–61]. This pattern is similar to what is seen with a left bundle branch block and is detrimental in terms of inotropy within the left ventricle [59]. Accordingly, any benefit from providing optimal LV preload by creating AV synchrony may be lost by the induction of dyssynchrony within the ventricles.

Treatment

A decision to refer for permanent pacemaker implantation for loss of atrioventricular synchrony due to first degree AV nodal block is challenging. In the setting of normal conduction in the ventricles, the improvement that may be gained by improving atrioventricular synchrony must be weighed against the dyssynchrony that may be caused by ventricular pacing. When ventricular dyssynchrony is already present, the decision becomes easier. Although some trials have demonstrated short-term hemodynamic benefits from AV optimization [51, 62, 63], others have not been able to demonstrate a benefit of AV optimization over empirically selecting a reasonable AV delay [53, 64]. This may be because the hemodynamic benefits that may be obtained occur at very short and very long AV delays, while any changes are modest for other AV delays [65].

Atrial Fibrillation and Heart Failure

Atrial fibrillation is commonly associated with heart failure, and the prevalence of atrial fibrillation is related to the severity of heart failure, with less than 5% affected with very mild heart failure to nearly 50% affected with advanced heart failure [66]. Heart failure and atrial fibrillation are both common cardiovascular disorders and share the same demographic risk factors, including age, history of hypertension, prior myocardial infarction, and valvular heart disease [67, 68]. Further, the incidence of heart failure increases dramatically after the diagnosis of atrial fibrillation [69]. Progression of LV dysfunction can clearly be associated with rapid ventricular rates [70–76]. Conversely, conversion to normal sinus rhythm or control of ventricular response in atrial fibrillation can improve LV function [71–74, 77]. Accordingly, rate control becomes very important in patients with heart failure and dilated cardiomyopathy, and likely even more so when ischemia from rapid rates complicate the patient's course.

Treatment

In patients with chronic heart failure, the use of digoxin and beta blockers is typically sufficient to control heart rates, and the combination of digoxin with carvedilol has been shown to provide better overall rate control than either of them used alone in heart failure patients [42]. However, if the patient is either intolerant of beta blockers or they fail to provide sufficient rate control, the next choice of treatment is less clear. The options are to add another drug, such as a calcium channel blocker or an antiarrhythmic drug that produces slowing of conduction within the AV node. However, both classes of drugs are associated with side effects or poor outcomes in heart failure. Accordingly, a rational strategy is to ablate the AV node and pace from the ventricles. This approach is very effective at providing rate control. However, the issue that follows is whether the benefit in terms of rate control outweighs the alteration in the normal activation of the ventricles induced with ventricular pacing.

Intraventricular Conduction System Disease

Intraventricular conduction system disease is associated with a number of poor prognostic indicators in heart failure, including LV size, ejection fraction, and severity of symptoms [1–3, 20, 78]. Further, within individual patients, progression of conduction system disease has been associated with progression of LV remodeling and worsening of heart failure [4]. Intraventricular conduction delays by definition create a delay in delivering the electrical wave of depolarization throughout the ventricles. The result is also a mechanical delay between both right and left ventricles, as well as a delay in mechanical activation between the portions of the left ventricle. This mechanical dyssynchrony has been measured in detail using a number of techniques including three-dimensional reconstruction of MRI images, gated radionuclide blood pool scanning, and several echocardiographic measurements [79–85]. Because of the wide availability, variety of measurements that can be made, along with advent of several newer techniques such as strain rate imaging, echocardiography has become the method of choice for demonstrating cardiac dyssynchrony.

Intraventricular conduction delay often leads to late activation of the left ventricular free wall with significant mechanical consequences. The mechanical consequences of abnormal electrical activation of the heart have long been recognized [58, 60, 86]. These include dyssynchrony between the atria,

inappropriate timing of atrial contribution to ventricular filling, timing delays between the ventricles that may have implications on septal motion and ventricular interdependence, and coordination of the left ventricle [87–89]. The wave of depolarization and mechanical activation have been studied in detail. Left bundle branch blocks produce a delay in conduction to the LV free wall [81]. The result is that the septum activates early and begins contraction against a low intraventricular pressure [90]. By the time activation begins in the LV free wall, the septum has completed much of its shortening against a low afterload, yet ejection is just beginning [91]. Additionally, the contraction of the septum prior to the initiation of contraction in the free wall of the left ventricle causes unusual stretch within the free wall just prior to the initiation of its contraction. The free wall is left with both an increase in preload, delivered to it by early contraction of the septum, as well as a high afterload, since the initiation of contraction occurs well into systole. Conversely, the early activated septum undergoes a late systolic, paradoxical stretch [82]. The result is an internal "sloshing" of blood from side to side within the left ventricle at the expense of forward stroke volume [91]. Additionally, the end-systolic stress is increased by the larger ventricular volume at end systole, and this is amplified in the free wall by the prolonged higher pressures during systole. Although this pattern is most evident in a typical left bundle branch block, many patients with heart failure have a nonspecific intraventricular conduction delay or a right bundle branch block [92]. Often in advanced ischemic heart failure, even with right bundle branch block, there is still a delay in electrical and mechanical activation of the LV free wall [93]. There are several studies that have demonstrated that the location of pacing has an influence on hemodynamics, and the right ventricular endocardium has not been one of the favored sites [58, 94].

Secondary mitral regurgitation can be a consequence of intraventricular conduction delay. Secondary mitral regurgitation is a common accompaniment of dilated cardiomyopathy of ischemic etiology. Intraventricular conduction delays can create or exacerbate mitral regurgitation by causing a lack of coordination of the papillary muscles [95]. The geometry of the mitral papillary muscles places one near the septum and one near the free wall. The same discoordination seen in wall motion leads to delays in contraction of the papillary muscles, and an increase in mitral regurgitation. Indeed, right ventricular pacing can acute cause mitral regurgitation by the change in the pattern of electrical depolarization [96–99]. This can be corrected with appropriately placed pacing leads and biventricular stimulation [47, 95, 100].

Intraventricular conduction delays cause diastolic dysfunction. Intraventricular conduction delays lead to a longer time period from the onset of depolarization within the ventricles to the ejection phase, as much of the ventricle must contract before ejection occurs [59]. Additionally, systole ends late with the segments depolarized late beginning relaxation late as well. The net result is prolonged isovolumic contraction time, delayed initiation of ejection, delayed initiation of relaxation, and prolonged isovolumic relaxation time. This leaves significantly less time during the cardiac cycle for diastole. In addition to the shortening of diastole, just as systole occurs in a discoordinate fashion, diastole also occurs slowly and discoordinately. The shortening of diastole along with the delay in relaxation in the ventricle contribute to the inefficiency of cardiac performance.

Metabolic and genetic effects of conduction system disease are associated with intraventricular conduction delays. The abnormal loading conditions induced by the discoordinate contraction of the ventricles leads to regional changes in myocardial perfusion, oxygen consumption, and may lead to differing hypertrophic responses within the ventricle [90, 101]. Studies have demonstrated that the oxygen consumption in the LV free wall is increased compared with the septum, and myocardial perfusion is also increased in the free wall [102]. However, in ischemic heart disease, the extent of coronary artery disease perfusing the free wall may limit the ability of the free wall to compensate for the increase in loading conditions. These abnormal loading conditions have now been shown in animal models to be associated with changes in gene expression, or remodeling of the myocardium on a molecular level [103]. In this study, a dog model of heart failure created by rapid-pacing from either the right atrium or the high right ventricular free wall. Right ventricular pacing was shown to create a markedly

dyssynchronous ventricular contraction. In the dyssynchronous hearts, the lateral LV endocardium displayed a twofold increase in phosphorylated *erk* mitogen-activated protein kinase expression, a 30% decrease in sarcoplasmic reticulum calcium-ATPase, an 80% reduction in phospholamban, and a 60% reduction in gap junction protein connexin 43 relative to neighboring myocardial segments. In contrast, the hearts from animals paced in the right atrium exhibited no such change in protein expression. This demonstrates the effect of mechanical dyssynchrony on protein expression, particularly within the late-activated lateral wall that has the greatest increase in loading conditions.

Energetics of the heart are adversely affected by intraventricular conduction delays. The inefficiency inherent in ventricular contraction with intraventricular conduction delays would be expected to produce an increase in energy expenditure that may be corrected with improving the mechanical coordination with biventricular stimulation. Indeed, this has been demonstrated in ten patients who have left bundle branch block and heart failure with dilated cardiomyopathy [104]. In this study, biventricular stimulation led to an $8 \pm 6.5\%$ decrease in myocardial oxygen consumption while providing a $43 \pm 6\%$ increase in dP/dt. Therefore, more force was generated with less energy requirements, a marked improvement in myocardial efficiency. This was compared with a similar degree of increased inotropy with dobutamine, which caused the expected $22 \pm 11\%$ increase in oxygen consumption.

Clinical Studies of Multisite Pacing

A series of pilot studies began with multisite pacing for patients with heart failure and dilated cardiomyopathy in the early 1990s [52, 105–111]. An improvement in LV function and symptoms of heart failure were demonstrated. This provided the interest in biventricular pacing for heart failure. The term cardiac resynchronization therapy was coined to refer to pacing therapies that attempt to enhance cardiac performance by using pacing to correct electrical conduction abnormalities in the heart. The most common form of this therapy is atrial-synchronous biventricular pacing. In this mode, atrial activation is sensed and triggers pacing in both ventricles. Early pilot studies utilized epicardial leads to access the left ventricle [106, 107]. However, an endovascular approach was developed by cannulating the coronary sinus and guiding pacing leads selectively into coronary veins in the LV free wall territory [109, 111]. By simultaneously stimulating the right ventricular endocardium and LV free wall epicardium, improved coordination between the ventricles and within the left ventricle is achieved.

Initial trials were pioneering in nature and attempted to demonstrate the effect, timing, and mechanisms [52, 106, 111, 112]. Later clinical trials were designed to more rigorously establish efficacy. A series of these later trials had a similar set of entry criteria that are summarized in Table 4.1 [113–116]. The criteria included a prolonged QRS duration, low ejection fraction, and advanced symptoms of heart failure. The baseline demographic features within these trials are displayed in Table 4.2. The features are consistent with a typical population with advanced heart failure. Importantly, the majority of the patients studied within these trials had ischemic heart disease as the etiology of heart failure. In each of the trials, the patient was first successfully implanted with a biventricular pacing device, and then randomized to months of pacing therapy on versus pacing therapy off. In the

MUSTIC trial, there was a 3-month study period followed by a crossover to the alternate pacing mode [113]. The patient was blinded to the treatment assignment, and the patient was assessed by blinded observers (creating a double-blind), although the physician and other medical personnel responsible for pacemaker function were by necessity unblinded to treatment assignment. The primary time point to establish efficacy was six months of pacing therapy. The metrics used included 6-min hall walk distance, NYHA functional class, global assessment, quality of life measures, and cardiopulmonary exercise testing. One trial had a primary endpoint of a composite of morbidity and mortality endpoints, but did not reach that endpoint because of a lower than expected incidence of these events. There was a consistent effect was seen in all heart failure measurements and the magnitude of benefit was clinically important (see Fig. 4.2) Although some of metrics used could be questioned because of the subjective nature of measurement and the possibility of unintentional unblinding, some of the metrics were more objective, such as peak oxygen consumption during cardiopulmonary exercise testing. In this metric, there was no evidence of a placebo effect, yet the treatment was associated with an increase in peak oxygen consumption greater than that typically seen in studies of pharmacologic agents [117]. These studies established

Table 4.1 Entry criteria in randomized trials of cardiac resynchronization therapy

	MUSTIC	MIRACLE	MIRACLE-ICD	CONTAK-CD
LVEF	<35%	≤35%	≤35%	≤35%
QRS duration	>150 ms	≥130 ms	≥130 ms	≥120 ms
NYHA class	III	III/IV	III/IV	II–IV*
LVIDD	>60 mm	≥55 mm	≥55 mm	–

*Although this study included patients with NYHA functional class II-IV heart failure, only those with NYHA functional class III-IV heart failure appeared to benefit. Subsequent graphics display only data from those with class III-IV heart failure at baseline.

Table 4.2 Baseline demographics in randomized trials of cardiac resynchronization therapy

	MUSTIC	MIRACLE	MIRACLE-ICD	CONTAK-CD
Number of Pts	67	453	362	490
Age	64 ± 10	65 ± 11	68 ± 10	66 ± 11
Gender (% male)	83	68	77	78
NYHA class (% III/IV)	100	91/9	89/11	89/11
LVEF (%)	23 ± 8	22 ± 6	20 ± 6	21 ± 6
Ischemic (%)	47	54	68	68
Peak VO_2 (ml/kg/min)	14.3 ± 4.0	14.3 ± 3.4	13.5 ± 3.9	12.0 ± 3.0
QRS duration (ms)	173 ± 18	166 ± 21	164 ± 22	158 ± 27

A. Effect of CRT on NYHA Functional Class

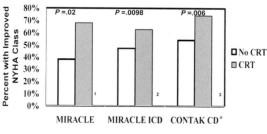

*- Class III/IV Patients

B. Effect of CRT on 6-minute Hall Walk Distance

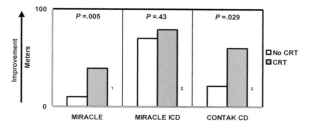

C. Effect of CRT on Peak Oxygen Consumption

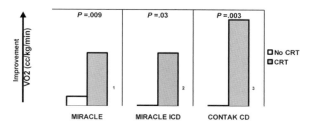

Fig. 4.2 In Panel **A**, the effects of CRT on NYHA class is shown for three trials, all of which shared similar entry criteria and a 6-month randomized, double-blind study duration. In each graphic, control (no CRT) is represent in *open boxes* and patient treated with CRT (CRT) in *hashed boxes*. Panel **B** represents the effect of CRT on 6-min hall walk distance and Panel **C** represents the peak oxygen consumption on cardiopulmonary exercise testing

the utility of biventricular pacing as a treatment for heart failure.

However, the long-term effects of cardiac resynchronization therapy (CRT) on morbidity and mortality were not known. Two clinical trials have established the morbidity and mortality effects of CRT. The COMPANION trial was a three armed trial, testing optimal medical therapy (OPT) against OPT plus CRT by a pacemaker or a OPT plus CRT by an implantable cardioverter-defibrillator (CRT-D) [118]. In this study, patients were enrolled prior to

implant, a true intent-to-treat design, and randomized in a 1:2:2 ratio to OPT, CRT, or CRT-D. The primary endpoint of the study was the combination of all cause mortality or all-cause hospitalization, with the highest order secondary endpoint being all-cause mortality. If a hospitalization was required for device implant, it was, by necessity, not counted as a primary endpoint. However, the primary endpoint did take into account competing risks of device implants, such as admissions for device revision, ICD shocks, and device infections. Enrollment was stopped when the anticipated number of primary endpoints was reached and at the same time, the pre-specified stopping criteria established by the Data Safety and Monitoring Board of the trial were reached. Both CRT and CRT-D treatments produced a 19–20% relative risk reduction in the primary endpoint (hazard ratio for CRT 0.81; $P = 0.014$; CRT-D 0.80; $P = 0.01$). CRT-D reduced mortality by 36% (hazard ratio 0.64; $P = 0.003$), while CRT trended toward a lower mortality with a 24% risk reduction (hazard ratio 0.76; $P = 0.059$). Along with the morbidity and mortality improvements, improvements in 6-min walk distance, quality of life measures and NYHA functional class were seen with both CRT and CRT-D that were consistent with prior studies.

There were problems with the COMPANION trial that related mainly to withdrawal of patients from the control group as CRT became available within the United States. As a result, more patients withdrew consent and were initially lost to follow-up in the OPT group (26%) as compared to either CRT or CRT-D groups (6–7%). As a result, a process of reconsent was established to gather primary endpoint and mortality data on patients who had withdrawn prior to a primary endpoint. After this process, primary endpoint status was known to 91% of the OPT group and 96% of the other two groups, while mortality data was complete in 96% of the OPT group and 99% of the CRT and CRT-D groups.

The CARE-HF study was a European study of medical therapy alone versus medical therapy with the addition of a CRT pacemaker [119]. A total of 813 patients were enrolled and randomized in a 1:1 ratio prior to device implant, again a true intent-to-treat design. Patients were followed longer than in the COMPANION trial, for a mean of 29.4 months. The primary end point was the time to death from any cause or an unplanned hospitalization for a major cardiovascular event. The first order secondary endpoint was all-cause mortality. The entry criteria were similar to other clinical trials of CRT, requiring a low ejection fraction, class III or IV heart failure, and a prolonged QRS duration. However, a second set of criteria was established for patients with a QRS duration between 120 and 149 ms in an attempt to demonstrate mechanical dyssynchrony. These patients were required to demonstrate two out of three criteria including an aortic pre-ejection period greater than 140 ms, and interventricular delay of greater than 40 ms, or delayed activation of the posterolateral wall.

In this study, CRT reduced the primary endpoint by 37% (hazard ratio 0.63; $P < 0.001$) and all-cause mortality by 36% (hazard ratio 0.64; $P < 0.001$). Although the relative risk reduction for mortality at first appears larger than that which trended in COMPANION (24% versus 36%), the mortality benefit was not evident in the early portion of the trial, but the benefit grew over time (see Fig. 4.3). Therefore, much, if not all, of the difference can be attributed to the longer follow-up (29.4 months in CARE-HF versus 14.8–16.5 months in COMPANION).

CRT is effective in patients with either ischemic or nonischemic dilated cardiomyopathy. The etiology of heart failure was not a predictor of outcomes in either the COMPANION trial or the CARE-HF trial [118, 119] (see Fig. 4.4). The trials were both performed in a broad range of patients with heart failure and low ejection fraction and the results appear to apply equally well to either those with or without ischemic disease. There have been some data that have suggested a differential effect of CRT based on etiology of heart failure. In general, these have been measures of reverse remodeling or the heart becoming smaller with a higher ejection fraction. St. John Sutton et al. reported better reverse remodeling in the MIRACLE trial for patients who had nonischemic dilated cardiomyopathy [120]. However, those with ischemic cardiomyopathy also had reverse remodeling, albeit to a lesser extent. Similar findings were seen in the CONTAK CD trial of biventricular pacing with an ICD [116]. In none of the trials were any clinical endpoints significantly associated with the etiology of heart failure. Therefore, the clinical implications of the studies appear to apply equally well to both nonischemic as well as ischemic dilated cardiomyopathy.

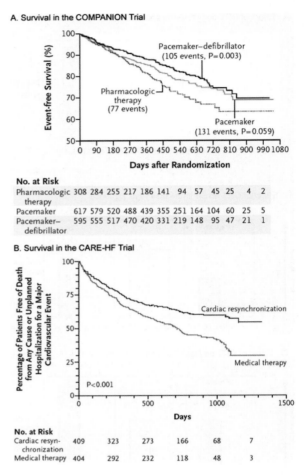

Fig. 4.3 Survival in the long-term randomized trials of CRT. In Panel **A**, the survival in the COMPANION trial was trended to improve by 24% in the cardiac resynchronization therapy (CRT) group ($P = 0.059$), but improved by 36% with CRT with ICD capability (CRT-D). Panel **B** shows the mortality results from the CARE-HF study. CRT reduced mortality by 36% with a longer follow-up than the COMPANION trial. Note that in both studies, the survival benefit CRT appears to increase with time

CRT promotes reverse remodeling. In addition to the clinically relevant endpoints in symptoms and functional capacity along with morbidity and mortality, the effects of CRT have been evaluated in several studies with echocardiography. These studies have consistently demonstrated benefit in reducing LV dimensions and increasing ejection fraction along with varied other measures of cardiac function including severity of mitral regurgitation, isovolumic contraction time, and measures of diastolic performance [93, 100, 114–116, 120–122].

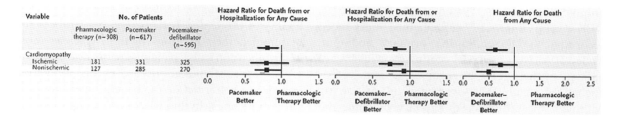

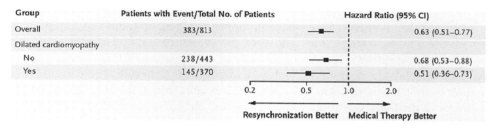

Fig. 4.4 Morbidity and mortality effects of CRT in ischemic and nonischemic cardiomyopathy. Panel **A** shows the effects of CRT and CRT-D on the primary endpoint of all-cause hospitalization and all-cause mortality, along with the effect of CRT-D on mortality for all patient, and patients with either ischemic or nonischemic cardiomyopathy. In Panel **B**, the effects of CRT on the primary endpoint of death or major cardiovascular hospitalization is shown for both ischemic and nonischemic cardiomyopathy

Treatment

CRT is now recommended for patients with LVEF less than or equal to 35%, sinus rhythm, and NYHA functional class III or ambulatory class IV symptoms despite recommended, optimal medical therapy and who have cardiac dyssynchrony, which is currently defined as a QRS duration greater than 0.12 ms, unless contraindicated. To date, over 4,000 patients have been studied in randomized clinical trials of CRT. A recent evaluation of complications from those studies suggest a risk of implant mortality of 0.4%, failure to implant a functioning LV lead in 10%, lead malfunction or dislodgement in 8.5%, and pacemaker infection in 1.4% [123].

CRT in Other Patient Populations

The effects of CRT in mild heart failure have not been established. There have been two large-scale trials that included patients with NYHA functional class II heart failure—the CONTAK CD trial and the MIRACLE ICD trial [115, 116]. Although there was no consistent clinical benefit seen in either trial, both studies revealed evidence of reverse

remodeling. Since these patients had only a modest degree of symptoms, improvements in these metrics are not as critical as it is for more advanced heart failure. Rather, the goal in such patients is to slow the progression of heart failure and avoid future morbidity and mortality. There are now two long-term randomized clinical trials evaluating the effects of biventricular pacing in mild heart failure—the REVERSE trial and the MADIT-CRT trial. Results of the REVERSE trial were recently published [140]. The REVERSE trial enrolled 684 patients with Class I (previously symptomatic) or II heart failure, a prolonged QRS duration (>120 ms), a low ejection fraction (LVEF ≤ 40%), and LV end diastolic diameter ≥ 55 mm. Permanent cardiac pacing was not permitted, but patients could enroll with or without an ICD indication. In this study, all patients received a CRT device (with or without ICD function as per current guidelines) and they were randomized to CRT on or off for the first year, followed by CRT off. The primary endpoint of this study was a heart failure clinical composite response describing the patient as improved, unchanged, or worsened based on symptoms, clinical events, and LV remodeling. A secondary endpoint compared left ventricular end systolic volume index (LVESVi) in the CRT OFF and CRT ON groups. At 12 months, 79% of patients in the CRT OFF group improved or remained unchanged according to the composite primary endpoint, while 21% worsened. By comparison, 84% of patients in the CRT ON group were improved or unchanged, and 16% worsened ($P = 0.10$). Although the difference in primary outcome did not reach statistical significance, the CRT did appear to reduce LV remodeling in this patient population. At 12 months, the LVESVi was decreased by 1.3 ml/m^2 and 18.4 ml/m^2 in the CRT OFF and CRT ON groups, respectively ($P < 0.0001$). CRT was also able to delay HF hospitalizations by 53%. The time to first HF hospitalization was significantly longer in the CRT ON compared with the CRT OFF group (Hazard Ratio, 0.47; $P = 0.03$). The blinded phase of REVERSE will continue for a total of 24 months, at which time additional data on clinical outcome, LV remodeling, and healthcare utilization will be available.

The MADIT-CRT trial is enrolling patients who have an indication for an ICD, a low ejection fraction (LVEF $\leq$ 40%), Class I or II heart failure, and a prolonged QRS duration to either an ICD alone or a CRT-D device. The primary endpoint of this study is all-cause mortality.

The effects of CRT in patients who are already pacemaker dependent have not been established in a randomized clinical trial. Randomized trials of CRT excluded patients who had an indication for permanent pacing. This was necessary for the double-blind assignment to pacing on or off. However, right ventricular pacing causing an electrical depolarization and a mechanical activation that is very similar to that seen in a patient with a left bundle branch block [90]. Accordingly, it is intuitive that such patients could benefit from CRT as opposed to right ventricular pacing. There was one randomized study reported that compared the right ventricular to biventricular pacing. However, the patient population was very different from that seen in other clinical trials of CRT. Patients with atrial fibrillation who were referred for AV nodal ablation for control of the rate response were enrolled in the study and randomized to either right ventricular or biventricular pacing after AV nodal ablation [124]. The majority of the patients were either NYHA class I or II and the mean LVEF was 46%. After 6 months of pacing therapy, patients randomized to

biventricular pacing had fewer symptoms, better quality of life scores, better exercise tolerance, and maintained their ejection fraction, whereas those with right ventricular pacing experienced a drop in LVEF. More studies are needed in this population in order to better define the benefit, particularly in patients in sinus rhythm with more severe disease.

Who responds well to CRT? An area of great interest in pacing for heart failure is that not all patients appear to benefit following initiation of CRT [80, 88, 89, 93, 125–128]. Given the cost and complexity of implantation of these devices, a very high rate of benefit is desirable. The percentage of patients who benefit from CRT is generally quoted between 50 and 80%. The variability in this assessment likely depends greatly on the specific metric used to define a patient as having responded beneficially to the therapy. Currently, there is no widely accepted definition of appropriate response to CRT therapy. Since symptoms are often improved in patients in the control arm of CRT trials, symptoms may not represent the most precise way of defining response. Cardiopulmonary exercise testing is not performed in routine clinical practice, and may not necessarily correlate with a symptomatic improvement. Some have proposed evidence of reverse remodeling as the appropriate way of identifying responders. The advantage is that the measurements are objective and are often obtained in clinical practice. However, the type of echocardiographic measurements carefully made in clinical trials are not routinely made in clinical practice, and the anticipated improvement (3–5% increase in ejection) may be measurable in a population in a clinical trial, but falls within the usual error of measurement for an individual.

Finally, there is variability of the treatment given and the underlying disease process for any individual patient. For example, a patient may have substantial ventricular mechanical dyssynchrony and have a successfully placed CRT device with appropriate lead locations. If very careful measures of ventricular performance are made, the patient's heart functions better with CRT on than off. However, if the patient suffers from a subsequent myocardial infarction or progressive ischemia, he may not improve clinically. Accordingly, at the end of a trial period, such a patient is termed a nonresponder even though he may be doing better with the device than he would have without the device. Similarly, in any group of patients, some improve in the course of the clinical trial, and this improvement may take one of many forms including reverse remodeling. Even if such a patient had an implant that provided no apparent benefit, he would be termed a responder. Accordingly, it is very challenging to define response or lack of response within a clinical trial. Attempts at defining responders and nonresponders with pharmacologic therapy in heart failure have been tried, but because of only a modest specificity have not led to a process of selection of some patients with heart failure over others [129–132]. It is not clear at this time whether the same challenges will be seen with CRT.

However, the goal is to select patients most likely to benefit from therapy. In this aspect, some measures do tend to stand out. QRS duration seems to provide a consistent trend in multiple trials, with more beneficial response in those with the longest QRS durations [88, 89, 125]. QRS duration is clearly associated with the severity of mechanical dyssynchrony, and improving mechanical dyssynchrony is believed to be the mechanism by which CRT improves outcomes in heart failure. Accordingly, the goal is to identify and quantitate mechanical dyssynchrony to better define patients who are likely to improve with CRT. There currently is no accepted standard for the assessment of cardiac dyssynchrony. The CARE-HF trial used three metrics that either identify or have been associated with mechanical dyssynchrony [119, 120]. The use of tissue Doppler and strain-rate imaging created tremendous interest and research [80, 85, 133]. Although there are several small studies that have correlated some measure of patient outcome to the degree of mechanical dyssynchrony, this has not been studied in a large scale, multi-center format. Additionally, QRS duration has been the sole measure of dyssynchrony used for all large-scale trials, with the exception of a small percentage of patients in the CARE-HF trial. Accordingly, almost all the clinical trial experience rests solely on QRS duration. Although entry criteria for the clinical trials generally had a cutoff in the range of 120–130 ms, the vast majority of the patients in clinical trials of CRT had QRS durations in excess of 150 ms. Accordingly, we are confident in the clinical effects of CRT only in patients with very long QRS

duration. This is important because demographically, there are more patients with a QRS duration between 120 and 149 ms than there are greater than 150 ms [134]. The clinical response to CRT in the group of patients with a QRS duration between 120 and 149 ms may not be as robust as that seen with longer QRS durations. Further, several small clinical trials suggest that there are a substantial number of patients with "normal" QRS durations (<120 ms) who have mechanical dyssynchrony and appear to respond to biventricular pacing. Accordingly, there is a need to better define the patient population who will benefit from CRT, particular in those QRS duration less than 150 ms.

Finally, the response to CRT is also dependent on location of the pacing leads. Inter-atrial conduction delays can be large in patients with heart failure, particularly when pacing from the most common atrial location, the right atrial appendage. Pacing from the inter-atrial septum seems to minimize the delay between atria and shorten the timing between atrial stimulation mechanical activation of the left atrium [134]. The location of the right ventricular lead is also debated [135–138]. There are several small studies demonstrating a mechanical advantage to pacing from high in the right ventricular septum compared with right ventricular apex for biventricular pacing. However, the majority of the patients in the randomized clinical trials were paced from the right ventricular apex and still appeared to have a robust response.

The most technically challenging lead to place is the LV lead. Successful implant in clinical trials is typically accomplished 90% of the time, but this leaves a significant failure rate [113–115, 118, 119]. The failure rate seems to be decreasing with time as operators become more experienced and the tools for implanting the leads are improving. However, even with a successful implant, the precise target and the ability to get there are often not known. Acute hemodynamic studies have suggested that the target location for LV pacing is the middle of the LV free wall for most, but not all, patients [139]. However, in clinical trials, operator descriptions of lead location (anterior, lateral, posterior) do not seem to correlate well with clinical response. This may be a problem with either the imprecision of the description of the lead location, the inherent "noise" in the measurement being made, or variability between patients as to the ideal location of the lead. One might think that an ideal pacing system would allow the user to noninvasively reprogram the lead to stimulate at different locations, and then a non-invasive metric could be used to assess hemodynamic response. This is clearly a desirable goal, but for now the target location is the mid-lateral wall of the left ventricle, while being limited by the coronary venous anatomy in a given patient.

Chapter Summary

The cardiac conduction system is often diseased in advanced ischemic heart disease. Studies in the past decade have demonstrated both beneficial and detrimental effects of pacing in patients with chronic heart failure. We have learned the detrimental effects of causing a discoordinate contraction with right ventricular pacing, and the beneficial effects of improving the coordination of contraction with CRT in appropriately selected patients. Although sinus node dysfunction is a typical complication of heart failure and the pharmacologic treatment of heart failure exacerbates sinus node dysfunction, it is not clear when and how we should increase the atrial rate in patients with chronic heart failure. Although much has been learned recently and pacing therapy is now a standard treatment for advanced heart failure, much more information is needed about how and when to pace.

References

1. Baldasseroni S, Opasich C, Gorini M, et al. Left bundle-branch block is associated with increased 1-year sudden and total mortality rate in 5517 outpatients with congestive heart failure: a report from the Italian network on congestive heart failure. Am. Heart J. 2002;143:398–405.
2. Shamim W, Francis DP, Yousufuddin M, et al. Intraventricular conduction delay: a prognostic marker in chronic heart failure. Int. J. Cardiol. 1999;70:171–8.
3. Xiao HB, Roy C, Fujimoto S, Gibson DG. Natural history of abnormal conduction and its relation to prognosis in patients with dilated cardiomyopathy. Int. J. Cardiol. 1996;53:163–70.
4. Shamim W, Yousufuddin M, Cicoria M, Gibson DG, Coats AJ, Henein MY. Incremental changes in QRS duration in serial ECGs over time identify high risk elderly patients with heart failure. Heart 2002;88:47–51.
5. Benditt DG, Sakaguchi S, Goldstein MA, et al. Sinus node dysfunction, pathophysiology, clinical features, evaluation, and treatment. In: Zipes DP, Jalife J, eds. Cardiac electrophysiology: from cell to bedside. 2nd ed. Philadelphia: WB Saunders, 1995:1215–47.
6. Gomes JA, Winters SL, Stewart D, Horowitz S, Milner M, Barreca P. A new noninvasive index to predict sustained ventricular tachycardia and sudden death in the first year after myocardial infarction: based on signal-averaged electrocardiogram, radionuclide ejection fraction and Holter monitoring. J. Am. Coll. Cardiol. 1987;10:349–57.
7. Becker AE. Relationship between structure and function of the sinus node: general comments. In: Bonke FI, ed. The sinus node. The Hague: Martinus Nijhoff, 1978:212–22.
8. Hecht HH, Kossmann CE, Childers RW, et al. Atrioventricular and intraventricular conduction. Revised nomenclature and concepts. [Review, 68 refs]. Am. J. Cardiol. 1973;31:232–44.
9. Scherlag BJ, Lazzara R, Helfant RH. Differentiation of "A-V junctional rhythms". Circulation 1973;48:304–12.
10. James TN. Anatomy of the coronary arteries. New York: Hoeber, Harper & Row, 1961.
11. Rosenbaum M, Elizari MV, Lazzari JO. The Hemiblocks. Tampa: Tampa Tracings, 1970.
12. Demoulin JC, Kulbertus HE. Histopathological examination of concept of left hemiblock. Br. Heart J. 1972;34:807–14.
13. Uhley HN. Some controversy regarding the peripheral distribution of the conduction system. Am. J. Cardiol. 1972;30:919–20.
14. Godman MJ, Lassers BW, Julian DG. Complete bundle-branch block complicating acute myocardial infarction. N. Engl. J. Med. 1970;282:237–40.
15. Hindman MC, Wagner GS, JaRo M, et al. The clinical significance of bundle branch block complicating acute myocardial infarction. 1. Clinical characteristics, hospital mortality, and one-year follow-up. Circulation 1978;58:679–88.
16. Hindman MC, Wagner GS, JaRo M, et al. The clinical significance of bundle branch block complicating acute myocardial infarction. 2. Indications for temporary and permanent pacemaker insertion. Circulation 1978;58:689–99.
17. Scheinman MM, Gonzalez RP. Fascicular block and acute myocardial infarction. JAMA 1980;244:2646–9.
18. Sugiura T, Iwasaka T, Hasegawa T, et al. Factors associated with persistent and transient fascicular blocks in anterior wall acute myocardial infarction. Am. J. Cardiol. 1989;63:784–7.
19. Goldberg RJ, Zevallos JC, Yarzebski J, et al. Prognosis of acute myocardial infarction complicated by complete heart block (the Worcester Heart Attack Study). Am. J. Cardiol. 1992;69:1135–41.
20. Newby KH, Pisano E, Krucoff MW, Green C, Natale A. Incidence and clinical relevance of the occurrence of

bundle-branch block in patients treated with thrombolytic therapy. Circulation 1996;94:2424–8.

21. Stenestrand U, Tabrizi F, Lindback J, Englund A, Rosenqvist M, Wallentin L. Comorbidity and myocardial dysfunction are the main explanations for the higher 1-year mortality in acute myocardial infarction with left bundle-branch block. Circulation 2004;110:1896–902.

22. Sanders P, Morton JB, Davidson NC, et al. Electrical remodeling of the atria in congestive heart failure: electrophysiological and electroanatomic mapping in humans. Circulation 2003;108:1461–8.

23. Sanders P, Kistler PM, Morton JB, Spence SJ, Kalman JM. Remodeling of sinus node function in patients with congestive heart failure: reduction in sinus node reserve. Circulation 2004;110:897–903.

24. Nagele H, Bohlmann M, Eck U, Petersen B, Rodiger W. Combination therapy with carvedilol and amiodarone in patients with severe heart failure. Eur. J. Heart Fail. 2000;2:71–9.

25. Hilgard J, Ezri MD, Denes P. Significance of ventricular pauses of three seconds or more detected on twenty-four-hour Holter recordings. Am. J. Cardiol. 1985;55:1005–8.

26. Mazuz M, Friedman HS. Significance of prolonged electrocardiographic pauses in sinoatrial disease: sick sinus syndrome. Am. J. Cardiol. 1983;52:485–9.

27. Moss AJ, Zareba W, Hall WJ, et al. Prophylactic implantation of a defibrillator in patients with myocardial infarction and reduced ejection fraction. N. Engl. J. Med. 2002;346:877–83.

28. Bardy GH, Lee KL, Mark DB, et al. Amiodarone or an implantable cardioverter-defibrillator for congestive heart failure. N. Engl. J. Med. 2005;352:225–37.

29. Gregoratos G, Abrams J, Epstein AE, et al. ACC/AHA/NASPE 2002 guideline update for implantation of cardiac pacemakers and antiarrhythmia devices—summary article: a report of the American College of Cardiology/American Heart Association Task Force on Practice Guidelines (ACC/AHA/NASPE Committee to Update the 1998 Pacemaker Guidelines). J. Am. Coll. Cardiol. 2002;40:1703–19.

30. Wilkoff BL, Cook JR, Epstein AE, et al. Dual-chamber pacing or ventricular backup pacing in patients with an implantable defibrillator: the Dual Chamber and VVI Implantable Defibrillator (DAVID) Trial. [see comment]. JAMA 2002;288:3115–23.

31. Anonymous. A trial of the beta-blocker bucindolol in patients with advanced chronic heart failure. [see comment]. N. Eng. J. Med. 2001;344:1659–67.

32. Packer M, Coats AJ, Fowler MB, et al. Effect of carvedilol on survival in severe chronic heart failure. [see comment]. N. Eng. J. Med. 2001;344:1651–8.

33. The MERIT-HF Study Group. Effect of metoprolol CR/XL in chronic heart failure: Metoprolol CR/XL Randomised Intervention Trial in Congestive Heart Failure (MERIT-HF). Lancet 1999; 353: 2001–7.

34. CIBIS II Investigators and Committee. The cardiac insufficiency bisoprolol study II (CIBIS-II): a randomised trial. Lancet 1999; 353: 9–13.

35. Nagatsu M, Spinale FG, Koide M, et al. Bradycardia and the role of beta-blockade in the amelioration of left ventricular dysfunction. Circulation 2000;101:653–9.

36. Mulder P, Barbier S, Chagraoui A, et al. Long-term heart rate reduction induced by the selective I(f) current inhibitor ivabradine improves left ventricular function and intrinsic myocardial structure in congestive heart failure. Circulation 1674;109:1674–9.

37. Wannenburg T, Schulman SP, Burkhoff D. End-systolic pressure-volume and MVO2-pressure-volume area relations of isolated rat hearts. Am. J. Physiol. 1992;262:H1287–93.

38. Weiss RG, Gerstenblith G, Bottomley PA. ATP flux through creatine kinase in the normal, stressed, and failing human heart. Proc. Natl. Acad. Sci. U. S. A. 2005;102:808–13.

39. Burkhoff D, Weiss RG, Schulman SP, Kalil-Filho R, Wannenburg T, Gerstenblith G. Influence of metabolic substrate on rat heart function and metabolism at different coronary flows. Am. J. Physiol. 1991;261:H741–50.

40. Vallebona A, Gigli G, Orlandi S, Reggiardo G. Heart rate response to graded exercise correlates with aerobic and ventilatory capacity in patients with heart failure. Clin. Cardiol. 2005;28:25–9.

41. Auricchio A, Kloss M, Trautmann SI, Rodner S, Klein H. Exercise performance following cardiac resynchronization therapy in patients with heart failure and ventricular conduction delay. Am. J. Cardiol. 2002;89:198–203.

42. Agarwal AK, Venugopalan P. Beneficial effect of carvedilol on heart rate response to exercise in digitalised patients with heart failure in atrial fibrillation due to idiopathic dilated cardiomyopathy. Eur. J. Heart Fail. 2001;3:437–40.

43. Roche F, Pichot V, Da Costa A, et al. Chronotropic incompetence response to exercise in congestive heart failure, relationship with the cardiac autonomic status. Clin. Physiol. 2001;21:335–42.

44. Colucci WS, Ribeiro JP, Rocco MB, et al. Impaired chronotropic response to exercise in patients with congestive heart failure. Role of postsynaptic beta-adrenergic desensitization. Circulation 1989;80:314–23.

45. Hochleitner M, Hortnagl H, Ng CK, Gschnitzer F, Zechmann W. Usefulness of physiologic dual-chamber pacing in drug-resistant idiopathic dilated cardiomyopathy. [see comment]. Am. J. Cardiol. 1990;66:198–202.

46. Ishikawa T, Sumita S, Kimura K, et al. Prediction of optimal atrioventricular delay in patients with implanted DDD pacemakers. [see comment]. Pacing Clin. Electrophysiol. 1999;22:1365–71.

47. Nishimura RA, Hayes DL, Holmes DR, Jr., Tajik AJ. Mechanism of hemodynamic improvement by dual-chamber pacing for severe left ventricular dysfunction: an acute Doppler and catheterization hemodynamic study. J. Am. Coll. Cardiol. 1995;25:281–8.

48. Appleton CP, Basnight MA, Gonzalez MS. Diastolic mitral regurgitation with atrioventricular conduction abnormalities: relation of mitral flow velocity to transmitral pressure gradients in conscious dogs. J. Am. Coll. Cardiol. 1991;18:843–9.

49. Schnittger I, Appleton CP, Hatle LK, Popp RL. Diastolic mitral and tricuspid regurgitation by Doppler echocardiography in patients with atrioventricular block: new insight into the mechanism of atrioventricular valve closure. J. Am. Coll. Cardiol. 1988;11:83–8.

50. Panidis IP, Ross J, Munley B, Nestico P, Mintz GS. Diastolic mitral regurgitation in patients with atrioventricular conduction abnormalities: a common finding by Doppler echocardiography. J. Am. Coll. Cardiol. 1986;7:768–74.

51. Auricchio A, Sommariva L, Salo RW, Scafuri A, Chiariello L. Improvement of cardiac function in patients with severe congestive heart failure and coronary artery disease by dual chamber pacing with shortened AV delay. [see comment]. Pacing Clin. Electrophysiol. 1993;16:2034–43.

52. Auricchio A, Stellbrink C, Sack S, et al. The pacing therapies for congestive heart failure (PATH-CHF) study: rationale, design, and endpoints of a prospective randomized multicenter study. Am. J. Cardiol. 1999;83:11.

53. Gold MR, Feliciano Z, Gottlieb SS, Fisher ML. Dual-chamber pacing with a short atrioventricular delay in congestive heart failure: a randomized study. [see comment]. J. Am. Coll. Cardiol. 1995;26:967–73.

54. Gold MR, Shorofsky SR, Metcalf MD, Feliciano Z, Fisher ML, Gottlieb SS. The acute hemodynamic effects of right ventricular septal pacing in patients with congestive heart failure secondary to ischemic or idiopathic dilated cardiomyopathy. Am. J. Cardiol. 1997;79:679–81.

55. Saxon LA, Stevenson WG, Middlekauff HR, Stevenson LW. Increased risk of progressive hemodynamic deterioration in advanced heart failure patients requiring permanent pacemakers. Am. Heart J. 1993;125:1306–10.

56. Brecker SJ, Xiao HB, Sparrow J, Gibson DG. Effects of dual-chamber pacing with short atrioventricular delay in dilated cardiomyopathy. [see comment, erratum appears in Lancet 1992 Dec 12;340(8833): 1482]. Lancet 1992;340:1308–12.

57. Hochleitner M, Hortnagl H, Fridrich L, Gschnitzer F. Long-term efficacy of physiologic dual-chamber pacing in the treatment of end-stage idiopathic dilated cardiomyopathy. Am. J. Cardiol. 1992;70:1320–5.

58. Burkhoff D, Oikawa RY, Sagawa K. Influence of pacing site on canine left ventricular contraction. Am. J. Physiol. 1986;251:H428–35.

59. Xiao HB, Lee CH, Gibson DG. Effect of left bundle branch block on diastolic function in dilated cardiomyopathy. Br. Heart J. 1991;66:443–7.

60. Zile MR, Blaustein AS, Shimizu G, Gaasch WH. Right ventricular pacing reduces the rate of left ventricular relaxation and filling. J. Am. Coll. Cardiol. 1987;10:702–9.

61. Rosenqvist M, Bergfeldt L, Haga Y, Ryden J, Ryden L, Owall A. The effect of ventricular activation sequence on cardiac performance during pacing. Pacing Clin. Electrophysiol. 1996;19:1279–86.

62. Capucci A, Romano S, Puglisi A, et al. Dual chamber pacing with optimal AV delay in congestive heart failure: a randomized study. Europace 1999;1:174–8.

63. Alboni P, Scarfo S, Fuca G, Mele D, Dinelli M, Paparella N. Short-term hemodynamic effects of DDD pacing from ventricular apex, right ventricular outflow tract and proximal septum. G. Ital. Cardiol. 1998;28:237–41.

64. Gilligan DM, Sargent D, Ponnathpur V, Dan D, Zakaib JS, Ellenbogen KA. Echocardiographic atrioventricular interval optimization in patients with dual-chamber pacemakers and symptomatic left ventricular systolic dysfunction. Am. J. Cardiol. 2003;91:629–31.

65. Auricchio A, Stellbrink C, Block M, et al. Effect of pacing chamber and atrioventricular delay on acute systolic function of paced patients with congestive heart failure. The pacing therapies for congestive heart failure study group. The guidant congestive heart failure research group. Circulation 1999;99:2993–3001.

66. Maisel WH, Stevenson LW. Atrial fibrillation in heart failure: epidemiology, pathophysiology, and rationale for therapy. [Review, 48 refs]. Am. J. Cardiol. 2003;91:20.

67. Benjamin EJ, Levy D, Vaziri SM, D'Agostino RB, Belanger AJ, Wolf PA. Independent risk factors for atrial fibrillation in a population-based cohort. The Framingham heart study. JAMA 1994; 271: 840–4.

68. Kannel WB, D'Agostino RB, Silbershatz H, Belanger AJ, Wilson PW, Levy D. Profile for estimating risk of heart failure. Arch. Intern. Med. 1999; 159: 1197–204.

69. Wang TJ, Larson MG, Levy D, et al. Temporal relations of atrial fibrillation and congestive heart failure and their joint influence on mortality: the Framingham heart study. [see comment]. Circulation 2003; 107: 2920–5.

70. Bhagat K. Tachycardiomyopathy—a case report. Cent. Afr. J. Med. 1999; 45: 275–6.

71. Lazzari JO, Gonzalez J. Reversible high rate atrial fibrillation dilated cardiomyopathy. Heart 1997; 77: 486.

72. Kessler G, Rosenblatt S, Friedman J, Kaplinsky E. Recurrent dilated cardiomyopathy reversed with conversion of atrial fibrillation. Am. Heart J. 1997; 133: 384–6.

73. van den Berg MP, van Veldhuisen DJ, Crijns HJ, Lie KI. Reversion of tachycardiomyopathy after beta-blocker. Lancet 1667; 341: 26.

74. Kieny JR, Sacrez A, Facello A, et al. Increase in radionuclide left ventricular ejection fraction after cardioversion of chronic atrial fibrillation in idiopathic dilated cardiomyopathy. Eur. Heart J. 1992; 13: 1290–5.

75. Grogan M, Smith HC, Gersh BJ, Wood DL. Left ventricular dysfunction due to atrial fibrillation in patients initially believed to have idiopathic dilated cardiomyopathy. Am. J. Cardiol. 1570; 69: 1570–3.

76. Peters KG, Kienzle MG. Severe cardiomyopathy due to chronic rapidly conducted atrial fibrillation: complete recovery after restoration of sinus rhythm. Am. J. Med. 1988; 85: 242–4.

77. Manolis AG, Katsivas AG, Lazaris EE, Vassilopoulos CV, Louvros NE. Ventricular performance and quality of life in patients who underwent radiofrequency AV junction ablation and permanent pacemaker implantation due to medically refractory atrial tachyarrhythmias. J. Interv. Card. Electrophysiol. 1998; 2: 71–6.

78. Nielsen JC, Andersen HR, Thomsen PE, et al. Heart failure and echocardiographic changes during long-term follow-up of patients with sick sinus syndrome randomized to single-chamber atrial or ventricular pacing. Circulation 1998; 97: 987–95.

79. Mule JD, Martinelli F. Assessment of dyssynchrony in patients with severe heart failure by nuclear imaging: paradise lost and regained or lost and gone forever? [Review, 39 refs]. Ital. Heart J. 2005; 6: 96–105.

80. Notabartolo D, Merlino JD, Smith AL, et al. Usefulness of the peak velocity difference by tissue Doppler imaging technique as an effective predictor of response to cardiac resynchronization therapy. Am. J. Cardiol. 2004; 94: 817–20.

81. Sade LE, Kanzaki H, Severyn D, Dohi K, Gorcsan J, III. Quantification of radial mechanical dyssynchrony in patients with left bundle branch block and idiopathic dilated cardiomyopathy without conduction delay by tissue displacement imaging. Am. J. Cardiol. 2004; 94: 514–8.

82. Curry CW, Nelson GS, Wyman BT, et al. Mechanical dyssynchrony in dilated cardiomyopathy with intraventricular conduction delay as depicted by 3D tagged magnetic resonance imaging. Circulation 2000; 101: 4.

83. Kawaguchi M, Murabayashi T, Fetics BJ, et al. Quantitation of basal dyssynchrony and acute resynchronization from left or biventricular pacing by novel echocontrast variability imaging. J. Am. Coll. Cardiol. 2002; 39: 2052–8.

84. Kerwin WF, Botvinick EH, O'Connell JW, et al. Ventricular contraction abnormalities in dilated cardiomyopathy: effect of biventricular pacing to correct interventricular dyssynchrony. J. Am. Coll. Cardiol. 2000; 35: 1221–7.

85. Sogaard P, Egeblad H, Kim WY, et al. Tissue Doppler imaging predicts improved systolic performance and reversed left ventricular remodeling during long-term cardiac resynchronization therapy. J. Am. Coll. Cardiol. 2002; 40: 723–30.

86. Raichlen JS, Campbell FW, Edie RN, Josephson ME, Harken AH. The effect of the site of placement of temporary epicardial pacemakers on ventricular function in patients undergoing cardiac surgery. Circulation 1984;70:I118–23.

87. Cazeau S, Bordachar P, Jauvert G, et al. Echocardiographic modeling of cardiac dyssynchrony before and during multisite stimulation: a prospective study. Pacing Clin. Electrophysiol. 2003;26:137–43.

88. Nelson GS, Curry CW, Wyman BT, et al. Predictors of systolic augmentation from left ventricular preexcitation in patients with dilated cardiomyopathy and intraventricular conduction delay. Circulation 2000;101:2703–9.

89. Kass DA. Ventricular resynchronization: pathophysiology and identification of responders. [Review, 51 refs]. Rev. Cardiovasc. Med. 2003;4:S3–13.

90. Prinzen FW, Augustijn CH, Arts T, Allessie MA, Reneman RS. Redistribution of myocardial fiber strain and blood flow by asynchronous activation. Am. J. Physiol. 1990;259:H300–8.

91. Leclercq C, Kass DA. Retiming the failing heart: principles and current clinical status of cardiac resynchronization. [Review, 81 refs]. J. Am. Coll. Cardiol. 2002;39:194–201.

92. Galizio NO, Pesce R, Valero E, et al. Which patients with congestive heart failure may benefit from biventricular pacing? Pacing Clin. Electrophysiol. 2003;26:158–61.

93. Yu CM, Fung WH, Lin H, Zhang Q, Sanderson JE, Lau CP. Predictors of left ventricular reverse remodeling after cardiac resynchronization therapy for heart failure secondary to idiopathic dilated or ischemic cardiomyopathy. Am. J. Cardiol. 2003;91:684–8.

94. Tyers GF, Waldhausen JA. Effect of site of synchronous unipolar ventricular stimulation and volume loading on cardiac function. J. Surg. Res. 1973;15:271–84.

95. Kanzaki H, Bazaz R, Schwartzman D, Dohi K, Sade LE, Gorcsan J, III. A mechanism for immediate reduction in mitral regurgitation after cardiac resynchronization therapy: insights from mechanical activation strain mapping. J. Am. Coll. Cardiol. 2004;44:1619–25.

96. Berglund H, Nishioka T, Hackner E, et al. Ventricular pacing: a cause of reversible severe mitral regurgitation. Am. Heart J. 1996;131:1035–7.

97. Sassone B, De Simone N, Parlangeli G, Tortorici R, Biancoli S, Di Pasquale G. Pacemaker-induced mitral regurgitation: prominent role of abnormal ventricular activation sequence versus altered atrioventricular synchrony. Ital. Heart J. 2001;2:441–8.

98. Hanna SR, Chung ES, Aurigemma GP, Meyer TE. Worsening of mitral regurgitation secondary to ventricular pacing. J. Heart Valve Dis. 2000;9:273–5.

99. Cannan CR, Higano ST, Holmes DR, Jr. Pacemaker induced mitral regurgitation: an alternative form of pacemaker syndrome. Pacing Clin. Electrophysiol. 1997;20:735–8.

100. Linde C, Leclercq C, Rex S, et al. Long-term benefits of biventricular pacing in congestive heart failure: results from the MUltisite STimulation in cardiomyopathy (MUSTIC) study. [see comment]. J. Am. Coll. Cardiol. 2002;40:111–8.

101. Prinzen FW, Hunter WC, Wyman BT, McVeigh ER. Mapping of regional myocardial strain and work during ventricular pacing: experimental study using magnetic resonance imaging tagging. J. Am. Coll. Cardiol. 1999;33:1735–42.

102. Ukkonen H, Beanlands RS, Burwash IG, et al. Effect of cardiac resynchronization on myocardial efficiency and regional oxidative metabolism. [see comment]. Circulation 2003;107:28–31.

103. Spragg DD, Leclercq C, Loghmani M, et al. Regional alterations in protein expression in the dyssynchronous failing heart. Circulation 2003;108:929–32.

104. Nelson GS, Berger RD, Fetics BJ, et al. Left ventricular or biventricular pacing improves cardiac function at diminished energy cost in patients with dilated cardiomyopathy and left bundle-branch block. [erratum appears in Circulation 2001 Jan 23; 103 (3): 476]. Circulation 2000;102:3053–9.

105. Bakker PF, Meijburg HW, de Vries JW, et al. Biventricular pacing in end-stage heart failure improves functional capacity and left ventricular function. J. Interv. Card. Electrophysiol. 2000;4:395–404.

106. Auricchio A, Klein H. Multiple chambered pacing for treatment of congestive heart failure. Pacing Clin. Electrophysiol. 1995;18:750–1.

107. Cazeau S, Ritter P, Bakdach S, et al. Four chamber pacing in dilated cardiomyopathy. [see comment]. Pacing Clin. Electrophysiol. 1994;17:1974–9.

108. Cazeau S, Ritter P, Lazarus A, et al. Multisite pacing for end-stage heart failure: early experience. Pacing Clin. Electrophysiol. 1996;19:1748–57.

109. Daubert JC, Ritter P, Le Breton H, et al. Permanent left ventricular pacing with transvenous leads inserted into the coronary veins. Pacing Clin. Electrophysiol. 1998;21:239–45.

110. Leclercq C, Cazeau S, Le Breton H, et al. Acute hemodynamic effects of biventricular DDD pacing in patients with end-stage heart failure. J. Am. Coll. Cardiol. 1998;32:1825–31.

111. Leclercq C, Cazeau S, Ritter P, et al. A pilot experience with permanent biventricular pacing to treat advanced heart failure. [see comment]. Am. Heart J. 2000;140:862–70.

112. Stellbrink C, Breithardt OA, Franke A, et al. Impact of cardiac resynchronization therapy using hemodynamically optimized pacing on left ventricular remodeling in patients with congestive heart failure and ventricular conduction disturbances. [see comment]. J. Am. Coll. Cardiol. 2001;38:1957–65.

113. Cazeau S, Leclercq C, Lavergne T, et al. Effects of multisite biventricular pacing in patients with heart failure and intraventricular conduction delay. N. Engl. J. Med. 2001;344:873–80.

114. Abraham WT, Fisher WG, Smith AL, et al. Cardiac resynchronization in chronic heart failure. [see comment]. N. Engl. J. Med. 2002;346:1845–53.

115. Young JB, Abraham WT, Smith AL, et al. Combined cardiac resynchronization and implantable cardioversion defibrillation in advanced chronic heart failure: the MIRACLE ICD Trial. [see comment]. JAMA 2003;289:2685–94.

116. Higgins SL, Hummel JD, Niazi IK, et al. Cardiac resynchronization therapy for the treatment of heart failure in patients with intraventricular conduction delay and malignant ventricular tachyarrhythmias. [see comment]. J. Am. Coll. Cardiol. 2003;42:1454–9.

117. Cohn JN, Johnson G, Ziesche S, et al. A comparison of enalapril with hydralazine-isosorbide dinitrate in the treatment of chronic congestive heart failure. [see comment]. N. Engl. J. Med. 1991;325:303–10.

118. Bristow MR, Saxon LA, Boehmer J, et al. Cardiac-resynchronization therapy with or without an implantable defibrillator in advanced chronic heart failure. [see comment]. N. Engl. J. Med. 2004;350:2140–50.

119. Cleland JG, Daubert JC, Erdmann E, et al. The effect of cardiac resynchronization on morbidity and mortality in heart failure. N. Engl. J. Med. 2005;352:1539–49.

120. St John Sutton MG, Plappert T, Abraham WT, et al. Effect of cardiac resynchronization therapy on left ventricular size and function in chronic heart failure. [see comment]. Circulation 2003;107:1985–90.

121. Sogaard P, Kim WY, Jensen HK, et al. Impact of acute biventricular pacing on left ventricular performance and volumes in patients with severe heart failure. A tissue doppler and three-dimensional echocardiographic study. Cardiology 2001;95:173–82.

122. Lau CP, Yu CM, Chau E, et al. Reversal of left ventricular remodeling by synchronous biventricular pacing in heart failure. Pacing Clin. Electrophysiol. 2000;23:1722–5.

123. McAlister F, Ezekowitz J, Wiebe N, et al. Cardiac resynchronization therapy for congestive heart failure. Evid. Rep. Technol. Assess (Summ.) 2004;106:1–8.

124. Doshi RN. The left ventricular-based cardiac stimulation post av nodal ablation evaluation study. New Orleans, LA: American College of Cardiology Annual Scientific Sessions, 2004.

125. Molhoek SG, Van Erven L, Bootsma M, Steendijk P, Van Der Wall EE, Schalij MJ. QRS duration and shortening to predict clinical response to cardiac resynchronization therapy in patients with end-stage heart failure. Pacing Clin. Electrophysiol. 2004;27:308–13.

126. Oguz E, Dagdeviren B, Bilsel T, et al. Echocardiographic prediction of long-term response to biventricular pacemaker in severe heart failure. Eur. J. Heart Fail. 2002;4:83–90.

127. Reuter S, Garrigue S, Barold SS, et al. Comparison of characteristics in responders versus nonresponders with biventricular pacing for drug-resistant congestive heart failure. Am. J. Cardiol. 2002;89:346–50.

128. Yu CM, Zhang Q, Fung JW, et al. A novel tool to assess systolic asynchrony and identify responders of cardiac resynchronization therapy by tissue synchronization imaging. J. Am. Coll. Cardiol. 2005;45:677–84.

129. Schleman KA, Lindenfeld JA, Lowes BD, et al. Predicting response to carvedilol for the treatment of heart failure: a multivariate retrospective analysis. J. Card. Fail. 2001;7:4–12.

130. Lowes BD, Gill EA, Abraham WT, et al. Effects of carvedilol on left ventricular mass, chamber geometry, and mitral regurgitation in chronic heart failure. Am. J. Cardiol. 1201;83:1201–5.

131. Andersson B, Lomsky M, Waagstein F. The link between acute haemodynamic adrenergic beta-blockade and long-term effects in patients with heart failure. A study on diastolic function, heart rate and myocardial metabolism following intravenous metoprolol. Eur. Heart J. 1993;14:1375–85.

132. Groenning BA, Nilsson JC, Hildebrandt PR, et al. Neurohumoral prediction of left-ventricular morphologic response to beta-blockade with metoprolol in chronic left-ventricular systolic heart failure. Eur. J. Heart Fail. 2002;4:635–46.

133. Yu CM, Fung JW, Zhang Q, et al. Tissue Doppler imaging is superior to strain rate imaging and postsystolic shortening on the prediction of reverse remodeling in both ischemic and nonischemic heart failure after cardiac resynchronization therapy. [see comment]. Circulation 2004;110:66–73.

134. Shenkman HJ, Pampati V, Khandelwal AK, et al. Congestive heart failure and QRS duration: establishing prognosis study. Chest 2002;122:528–34.

135. Barin ES, Jones SM, Ward DE, Camm AJ, Nathan AW. The right ventricular outflow tract as an alternative permanent pacing site: long-term follow-up. Pacing Clin. Electrophysiol. 1991;14:3–6.

136. Buckingham TA, Candinas R, Attenhofer C, et al. Systolic and diastolic function with alternate and combined

site pacing in the right ventricle. Pacing Clin. Electrophysiol. 1998;21:1077–84.

137. Giudici MC, Thornburg GA, Buck DL, et al. Comparison of right ventricular outflow tract and apical lead
permanent pacing on cardiac output. Am. J. Cardiol.
1997;79:209–12.

138. Pachon JC, Pachon EI, Albornoz RN, et al. Ventricular endocardial right bifocal stimulation in the treatment of severe dilated cardiomyopathy heart failure
with wide QRS. Pacing Clin. Electrophysiol.
2001;24:1369–76.

139. Gold MR, Auricchio A, Hummel JD, et al. Comparison of stimulation sites within left ventricular
veins on the acute hemodynamic effects of cardiac
resynchronization therapy. Heart Rhythm
2005;2:376–81.

140. Linde C, Abraham WT, Gold MR, St John Sutton M,
Ghio S, Daubert C. Randomized trial of cardiac resynchronization in mildly symptomatic heart failure
patients and in asymptomatic patients with left ventricular dysfunction and previous heart failure symptoms.
J. Am. Coll. Cardiol. 2008;52:1834–43.

Chapter 5

The Role of Percutaneous Coronary Revascularization in Advanced Ischemic Heart Disease

Modern Angioplasty and Stent Technology; Technique, Application and Efficacy, Comparison to Surgical

Richard W. Smalling and Gregory M. Geisler

The only way to discover the limits of the possible is to go beyond them into the impossible.

Arthur C. Clarke

Historical Perspective

Coronary angiography and intervention has become the leading procedure to evaluate and treat coronary artery disease (CAD) with a history characterized by rapid evolution. It is remarkable that such a procedure began less than 40 years ago and continues to evolve (Fig. 5.1). Initiation of X-ray imaging, which has been instrumental to the practice of medicine, occurred in 1895 with Wilhelm Rontgen's first radiograph [1]. He found that an object (his wife's hand) exposed to an X-ray field could be imaged and captured on X-ray film. Improvements in imaging for diagnostic purposes flourished over the ensuing years. Early leaders of the interventional field took advantage of this technology, while going against the common beliefs of the time and some even risking their own lives to develop techniques to expand the field of cardiovascular medicine.

It was not until 1929 that the concept of central cardiac catheters came to being. Prior to this, it was felt that manipulation of the heart would lead to immediate death. Werner Forssmann, while a surgical fellow in Eberswald, Germany, believed there was a more efficient way to more rapidly administer medications. One night, in his office, he inserted a ureteral catheter into his own left basilic vein and walked upstairs to the radiology suite where he confirmed the location of the catheter in the right atrium. He was immediately fired and ostracized for his activities and further research over the next decade was limited. Then, in 1941, Andre Cournand and Dickinson Richards first described the use of catheterization as a diagnostic tool [2, 3]. For their efforts, these three pioneers received the 1956 Nobel Prize in Physiology or Medicine for "their discoveries concerning heart catheterization and pathologic changes in the circulatory system" [4] (Fig. 5.2).

The first diagnostic coronary angiogram was performed by Mason Sones, MD, a pediatric cardiologist at the Cleveland Clinic. While he was attempting to evaluate the aortic valve, contrast was injected through the catheter that had accidentally engaged the right coronary artery. The patient had no adverse event secondary to the injection and later Dr. Sones stated, "I knew that night that we finally had a tool that would define the anatomic nature of coronary artery disease" [5]. This led to the initial instrumentation of the coronary artery to define its anatomy and later as a therapeutic tool.

Until the early 1960s, the focus had been on diagnostic imaging and medication administration. Charles Dotter and Melvin Judkins turned the attention to therapeutic strategies [6–8]. Using

R.W. Smalling (✉)
Department of Internal Medicine-Cardiology, Medical
School Houston, University of Texas, Houston, TX, USA
e-mail: Richard.w.smalling@uth.tmc.edu

R. Delgado, H.S. Arora (eds.), *Interventional Treatment of Advanced Ischemic Heart Disease*,
DOI 10.1007/978-1-84800-395-8_5, © Springer-Verlag London Limited 2009

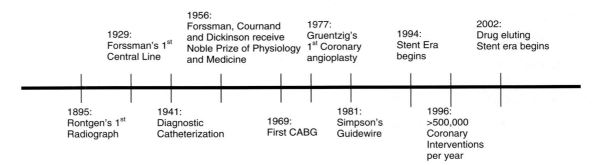

Fig. 5.1 Historical timeline of the coronary intervention evolution

the "Dottering" technique of back and forth manipulation, the catheter was used to open occluded peripheral arteries. There was a significant improvement in arterial flow; however, adverse events including access site bleeding and distal embolization limited overall success. In 1974, Andreas Gruentzig developed the first double lumen catheter with distal balloon, which, while inflated, shifted the plaque against the vessel wall. Procedural success of Gruentzig's technique was 86%.

Concurrently the philosophy of heart manipulation was also evolving. In 1969, Rene Favalaro et al. performed the first surgical coronary artery bypass grafting (CABG), launching the field of interventional techniques into the field of cardiovascular medicine [9]. Gruentzig, with this in mind, further refined the catheter with a smaller luminal diameter and in 1974 began coronary angioplasty studies in the animal and cadaveric model [10]. In May 1977, while in San Francisco, California, with the assistance of Richard Myler, the first coronary angioplasty in a live human was performed. This established the effects of angioplasty on the arterial lesion as well as the risk of distal embolization, which was

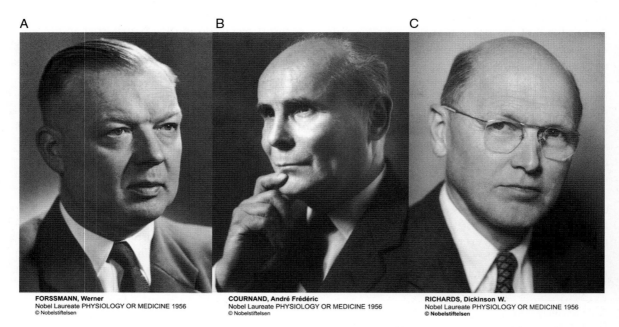

Fig. 5.2 1956 Noble Laureates of Physiology and Medicine: (**A**) Werner Forssman, (**B**) André Frédéric Cournand, (**C**) Dickinson W. Richards (© The Nobel Foundation)

not observed. Then in September of 1977, in Zurich, Gruentzig performed the first primary percutaneous transluminal coronary angioplasty (PTCA) in a catheterization laboratory [11]. Several years later, in 1981, John Simpson developed a through lumen PTCA balloon over a steerable guidewire. This technology led to PTCA of difficult to treat lesions and greatly expanded its utility [12]. One year later PTCA was used during the early treatment of acute myocardial infarction.

By 1996 over 500,000 coronary interventions were performed annually, which has more than doubled to today's current standard. These pioneers have paved the way for interventional procedures that now serve as the standard of care for symptomatic coronary artery disease. While coronary intervention remains in its adolescent stage, the quality of care has increased substantially and the bar is ever increasing as to the extent coronary interventions play in our society's healthcare.

PTCA Versus Medical Therapy with Stable Angina/Unstable Angina

The treatment of CAD for the alleviation of angina was evaluated in several trials that ultimately shaped the role of coronary angioplasty. Prior to this, trials such as the Veterans Administration Cooperative Study (VA Study) [13, 14] and the Coronary Artery Surgery Study (CASS) trial [15] established the role of revascularization for the improvement in survival and symptom relief. A meta-analysis (Table 5.1) regarding surgical revascularization (CABG) versus

medical therapy demonstrated a significant mortality reduction with CABG in patients with moderate to high risk (based on left ventricular function, coronary anatomy, and severity of ischemia) [16]. With the advent of PTCA, it was theorized that less invasive procedures could achieve similar results. However the majority of percutaneous interventions were completed on single vessel disease and showed no benefit in survival or freedom from myocardial infarction [17, 18]. In small trials (ACME and ACME 2), there was improvement in exercise time and quality of life (more profound in those with relief of angina); however, this decreased over time. RITA-2 (Randomized Intervention Treatment of Angina Trial), a large trial with higher risk cohort, confirmed these results with the early endpoint of death and non-fatal myocardial infarction higher in the interventional arm (6.3% versus 3.3%; $p = 0.02$) [19]. The Medicine, Angioplasty or Surgery Study (MASS) trial evaluated different treatment options for proximal LAD disease in patients with normal left ventricular function. The primary endpoint of death, myocardial infarction, and refractory angina at 3 years showed a marked benefit with CABG (using left internal mammary artery) with no difference between the medical and PTCA arm (3% versus 17 versus 24%, respectively) [20]. Both revascularization arms reduced exercise induced ischemia and symptoms, however, PTCA had an increase in the risk of future revascularization procedures.

PTCA versus traditional CABG in multi-vessel disease (2 or 3 vessel disease without left main disease) yielded similar results [21–23]. Invariably, overall survival and non-fatal myocardial infarction were similar; however, CABG provided more symptom

Table 5.1 Long-term mortality with CABG reperfusion versus medical therapy

Trial	N (Medical)	N (CABG)	5-year mortality (%) CABG/Med Tx.	7-year mortality (%) CABG/Med Tx.	10-year mortality (%) CABG/Med Tx.
VA	354	332	17.5/22.3	22.3/30	35.5/39.8
European	373	394	7.6/16	13/20.4	23.1/29.2
CASS	390	390	5.1/8.2	11/13.6	18.5/21.3
Texas	60	56	17.9/23	26.8/30	41.1/41.7
Oregon	49	51	7.8/15.7	13.7/22.4	27.4/28.6
New Zealand	49	51	9.8/13.7	13.7/26.5	29.4/32.7
New Zealand	50	50	16/16	20/22	34/32
Total	1,325	1,324	10.2/15.8 $p < 0.001$	15.8/21.7 $p < 0.001$	26.4/30.5 $p = 0.03$

Adapted from [16].

relief, likely from increased complete revascularization, and reduced future revascularization. The BARI trial demonstrated a marked benefit with CABG in the patients with diabetes mellitus. Five-year survival in those with diabetes mellitus who had CABG was significantly improved (80.6% versus 65.5%; $p = 0.003$), which continued through 7 years of follow-up (76.4% versus 55.7%; $p = 0.001$). This difference was not seen in those with no evidence of diabetes mellitus. PTCA achieved early symptom relief, increased exercise time, and enhanced quality of life scores. Due to procedural complications, patient characteristics, as well as the risk of re-stenosis, this decreased with time.

Several variables may increase restenosis including vascular recoil, microdissection, smooth muscle cell proliferation, remodeling, and thrombus formation [24]. The advent of the coronary stenting aimed to address this concern. Two trials landmark the coronary stent era: BENESTENT and STRESS [25, 26] (Table 5.2). In the BENESTENT trial (520 patients with single vessel CAD receiving percutaneous coronary intervention and stent placement (PCI) or PTCA for stable angina) the difference in event rates was heralded by a reduction in repeat procedures (relative risk, 0.58; 95% confidence interval, 0.40–0.85; $p = 0.005$) and rate of >50% restenosis at 7 month follow-up (22% versus 32% respectively; $p = 0.02$). The STRESS trial randomized 410 patients with symptomatic single vessel disease to receive the Palmaz-Schatz stent or PTCA with follow-up angiography at 6 months. Lesion success was higher in the stent arm (96.1% versus 89.6%; $p = 0.011$), had improved early luminal diameter (2.49 ± 0.43 mm versus 1.99 ± 0.47 mm; $p < 0.001$), and a reduction in restenosis (36.1% versus 42.1%; $p = 0.046$). Stent implantation

thus became a novel technique to address the Achilles' heel of traditional PTCA.

With growing enthusiasm of stent implantation, trials aimed to evaluate PCI versus CABG in multi-vessel disease. The Arterial Revascularization Therapies Study (ARTS) was the largest to evaluate revascularization strategies in the early stent era [27]; 1,205 patients with multi-vessel disease were randomized to PCI versus CABG with no difference in mortality, coronary, or cerbrovascular events at 1 year (PCI: 8.8% versus CABG: 9.3%). However in the PCI arm, 21% required repeat revascularization compared to 3.8% with CABG (RR 5.52). The secondary endpoint was 5-year adverse events. Again there was no difference in mortality (8.0% versus 7.8%; $p = 0.83$) or the combined endpoint of death, stroke, or myocardial infarction (PCI: 18.2% versus 14.9%; $p = 0.14$) [28]. Similar to 1-year results, need for repeat revascularization was considerably higher with bare metal stenting. While improved from prior PTCA trials, ARTS demonstrated that over time re-stenosis remained a significant burden of PCI.

The ERACI II trial enrolled a higher risk patient cohort including left main and proximal LAD disease [29]. Patients with multivessel disease amenable to either strategy were randomized to PCI (Gianturco-Roubin II) or CABG with the aim of complete revascularization. Primary endpoints of death, MI, stroke, or repeat revascularization at 30 days was likely to favor PCI do to the traditional early risk with CABG. PCI demonstrated a favorable outcome (3.6% versus 12.3%; $p = 0.002$) and reduced 30-day mortality (0.9% versus 5.7%; $p = 0.012$). While this was early, the ERACI II trial enrolled a higher risk patient population and demonstrated that PCI is at least as

Table 5.2 BENESTENT (7 month) and STRESS (6 month) follow up and angiographic results of PTCA and PCI

	Benstent PCI	Benestent PTCA	p	STRESS PCI	Stress PTCA	p
N	259	257		205	202	
MLD pre	1.07 ± 0.33	1.08 ± 0.31	NS	0.77 ± 0.27	0.75 ± 0.25	0.48
Post	2.48 ± 0.39	2.05 ± 0.33	<0.001	2.49 ± 0.43	1.99 ± 0.47	<0.001
f/u	1.82 ± 0.64	1.73 ± 0.55	0.09	1.56 ± 0.65	1.74 ± 0.60	0.007
Restenosis %	22	32	0.02	31.6	42.1	0.046
			RR (95% CI)			p
Mortality (%)	2 (0.8)	1 (0.4)	1.98	1.5	0	0.25
Repeat PTCA	26 (10)	53 (20.6)	0.49	11.2	12.4	0.72
MI	4 (1.6)	7 (2.7)	1.74	6.3	6.9	0.81
CABG	6 (2.3)	8 (3.1)	1.32	4.9	8.4	0.15

good as CABG in the short term. Similar to the ARTS trial, 5-year results were similar with regards to mortality and myocardial infarction; however, repeat revascularization was significantly higher in the PCI cohort. Additionally, at 5 years, there was a similar number of patients who remained asymptomatic or with Class I angina (PCI: 86% versus CABG: 92%; $p = 0.96$) [30].

Higher-risk patients such as those with unstable angina or non-ST-elevation myocardial infarction (NSTEMI) are at an increased risk of early adverse events. Thrombolytic therapy has demonstrated no benefit in clinical outcomes and in fact increases the risk of acute myocardial infarction [31–33]. Therapy, traditionally, has taken either a conservative approach with medical therapy and angiography reserved for recurrent signs of ischemia or an aggressive approach with early angiography and PCI. Trials originally showed contradictory results in the reduction of mortality with the aggressive approach [34–36]. The more recent Treat Angina with Aggrastat and determine Cost of Therapy with an Invasive or Conservative Strategy (TACTICS-TIMI 18) trial compared the two treatment strategies with glycoprotein IIb/IIIa inhibitor use included with early (<48 h) revascularization [37]. The primary endpoint of death, non-fatal myocardial infarction, and repeat hospitalization for recurrent ischemia at 6 months was improved with this aggressive approach (15.9% versus 19.4%; $p = 0.025$) (Fig. 5.3). The benefit was more profound with elevated biomarkers as opposed to normal Troponin T levels, which showed no difference. In evaluating this conflicting data, those at higher risk including elevated cardiac markers have more to gain with the aggressive approach. Treatment strategy must then be individually tailored based on cardiac risk score analysis.

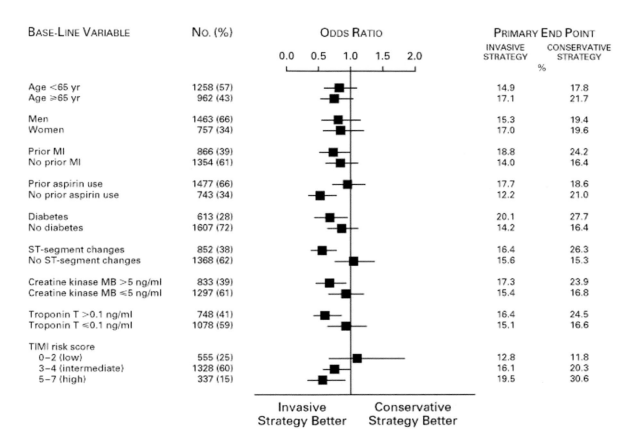

Fig. 5.3 Results of TACTICS TIMI 18. Primary end point of death, non-fatal myocardial infarction, and rehospitalization for acute coronary syndrome at 6 months based on baseline patient characteristics (© 2001 Massachusetts Medical Society)

Treatment of ST Elevation Myocardial Infarction

Initial trials with PCI focused on stable, symptomatic coronary artery disease and invariable excluded patients with an acute myocardial infarction (STEMI). Thrombolytic therapy provided early treatment for STEMI that could be used universally with a profound mortality benefit compared to conservative medical therapy. The Gruppo Italiano per lo Studio della Streptochinasi nell'Infarto Miocardico (GISSI) trial [38] demonstrated a reduction in 21 day mortality with streptokinase within 12 h of symptom onset (10.7% versus 13%; 18% reduction; $p = 0.0002$). In addition, earlier administration led to a further reduction in mortality, introducing an aggressive early treatment approach. International Study of Infarct Survival (ISIS-2) confirmed these findings and presented combination therapy including aspirin (ASA) as an added benefit [39]. Addition of ASA was superior to either therapy alone with reduced long term (median follow-up 15 months) death (8% versus 13.2%), reinfarction (1.85% versus 2.9%), as well as stroke (0.6% versus 1.1%).

While acute vessel patency improved, the benefits were not long standing. Three-month follow-up revealed a 32% risk of re-occlusion and 11% risk of reinfarction that was offset with ASA (Revascularization: 6% versus 16%; $p < 0.05$ and reinfarction: 3% versus 11%; $p < 0.025$) [40]. The benefit of thrombolysis given early had a profound outcome benefit; however, an increased risk of bleeding and since the plaque was not stabilized, a continued risk of reocclusion/reinfarction.

PTCA offered a different strategy to obtain vessel patency. Success rates were greater than 90% with low rates of bleeding and mortality [41, 42]. This was seen with both low in-hospital and 6 month mortality and reinfarction rate compared to thrombolysis (5.1% versus 12%; $p = 0.02$ and 8.5% versus 16.8%; $p = 0.02$, respectively) [43]. While there was no immediate benefit on ejection fraction, a similar study comparing PTCA with streptokinase showed a significant improvement in LVEF at the time of discharge with early PTCA (51 ± 11 versus 45 ± 12; $p = 0.004$) [44].

Obstacles remained as PTCA was not universally available and often associated with considerable time delay, especially in off peak hours. In the National Registry of Myocardial Infarction-2 (NRMI-2; >27,000 patients), total ischemia time (symptom onset to balloon inflation) was 3.9 h with onset to hospital arrival 1.6 h [45]. Unadjusted in-hospital mortality was higher in patients treated later. Door to balloon time > 2 h was related to in-hospital death (41–62% adjusted odds increase) and centers who treat >3 STEMIs/month had improved in-hospital mortality compared to less experienced facilities (Figs. 5.4 and 5.5). Lastly, similar to trials of unstable angina, PTCA was plagued by high restenosis rates

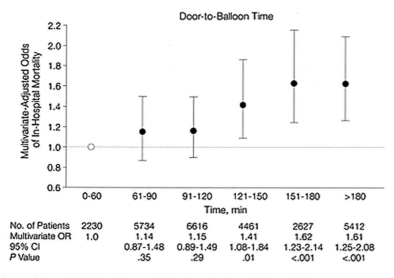

Fig. 5.4 NRMI database of door to balloon time as indicator of in-hospital mortality

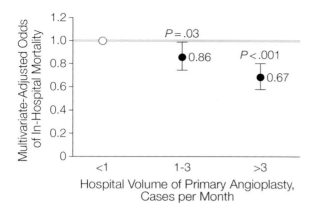

Fig. 5.5 In-hospital mortality compared with hospital volume in the NRMI database. Cannon: JAMA, Volume 283(22). June 14, 2000. 2941–2947

with a 43% angiographic restenosis and 14% reocclusion rate [46].

Stent therapy in STEMI remained intriguing because it allows for establishment of vessel patency and the ability to protect the culprit lesion. Several trials evaluated PCI versus PTCA, all showing a marked benefit in the combined endpoints of mortality and the requirement of revascularization with stenting [47–49]. The STENT PAMI trial helped shape the future of STEMI treatment. Overall mortality was not significantly different between the two groups; however, the combined end point of mortality, reinfarction, stroke, or revascularization was positive at 6 months owing to a marked increase in the requirement for revascularization in the PTCA

group (7.7% versus 17%; $p < 0.001$ and combined endpoint: 12.6% versus 20.1%; $p < 0.01$).

Interestingly, PCI had lower rates of normal flow (TIMI 3) compared to the angioplasty cohort. While this did not change clinical outcomes, it demonstrated the risk of distal embolization and no-reflow with stent implantation, marking the new era of glycoprotein IIb/IIIa inhibitors. Abciximab (a monoclonal Glycoprotein IIb/IIIa antibody) was associated with a reduced composite endpoint of death, reinfarction, and revascularization at 30 days (4.5% versus 26.1% placebo; $p = 0.06$) and at 6 months (4.5% versus 47.8%; $p = 0.002$); however, it did show a non-significant trend to higher major bleeding [50]. The **ADMIRAL** trial confirmed the benefit of pre-interventional use of abciximab. Thirty-day and six-month composite endpoints again were significantly improved with the inclusion of abciximab (30-day: 6% versus 14%; $p = 0.01$ and 6 month: 7.4% versus 15.9%; $p = 0.02$). In addition, there was marked improvement in normal TIMI 3 coronary flow on the initial angiogram (16.8% versus 5.4%; $p = 0.01$), post procedure (95.1% versus 86.7%; $p = 0.04$) and 6-month follow-up angiography (94.3% versus 82.8%; $p = 0.04$). Early PCI combined with glycoprotein IIb/IIIa inhibitors improved lumen patency, reduced thrombus burden, and improved coronary flow leading to increased myocardial salvage and thus reduced infarct size by technetium-99 myocardial perfusion imaging infarct size at 10 days. This approach has revolutionized the standard of care for STEMI, however, due to limited

Table 5.3 ACC/AHA 2004 executive summary guidelines for emergent PCI in STEMI

If immediately available, primary PCI should be performed in patients with STEMI (including true posterior MI) or MI with new or presumably new LBBB who can undergo PCI of the infarct artery within 12 h of symptom onset, if performed in a timely fashion (balloon inflation within 90 min of presentation) by persons skilled in the procedure (individuals who perform more than 75 PCI procedures per year). The procedure should be supported by experienced personnel in an appropriate laboratory environment (a laboratory that performs more than 200 PCI procedures per year, of which at least 36 are primary PCI for STEMI, and has cardiac surgery capability). (*Level of Evidence: A*)

Primary PCI should be performed for patients less than 75 years old with ST elevation or LBBB who develop shock within 36 h of MI and are suitable for revascularization that can be performed within 18 h of shock unless further support is futile because of the patient's wishes or contraindications/unsuitability for further invasive care. (*Level of Evidence: A*)

If symptom duration is greater than 3 h, primary PCI is generally preferred and should be performed with a medical contact-to-balloon or door-to-balloon interval as short as possible and a goal of within 90 min. (*Level of Evidence: B*)

If the symptom duration is within 3 h and the expected door-to-balloon time minus the expected door-to-needle time is within 1 h, primary PCI is generally preferred. (*Level of Evidence: B*)

Primary PCI should be performed in patients with severe CHF and/or pulmonary edema (Killip class 3) and onset of symptoms within 12 h. The medical contact-to-balloon or door-to-balloon time should be as short as possible (i.e., goal within 90 min). (*Level of Evidence: B*)

staffing and availability of 24 h high volume centers, many patients are not able to receive this approach. The ACC/AHA guidelines on acute STEMI emphasize the importance of early recognition and prompt initiation of reperfusion strategies, with PCI indicated in experienced institutions and operators who have a door to balloon time within 90 min. In addition primary PCI is preferred in patients presenting with cardiogenic shock or significant congestive heart failure [51] (Table 5.3).

Drug Eluting Stent Era

With the expansion of PCI, focus shifted to address the issue of in-stent restenosis. Applications in high risk sub-groups including those with diabetes mellitus, small vessel size, and longer lesions pushed the restenosis rate to nearly 30% [52–54]. While systemic therapy was not promising, utilization of drug-coated stents that would deliver anti-proliferative agents directly to the site of implantation was intriguing.

Rapamycin (sirolimus), a macrolide antibiotic, has been used recently in organ transplantation for its potent immunosuppressive actions by inhibiting both cytokine mediated and growth factor mediated proliferation of smooth muscle cells and lymphocytes [55, 56]. In the RAVEL trial of non-acute single vessel lesions, the Sirolimus-eluting stent was compared to bare metal stent (BMS) in a 1:1 fashion [57]. One-year major adverse cardiovascular events and 6 month neointimal proliferation as assessed by late luminal loss (-0.01 ± 0.33 mm in Sirolimus stent versus 0.80 ± 0.53 mm in BMS) were improved. The Sirolimus-eluting stent thus virtually eliminated in-stent restenosis with no evidence of edge effect, dissection, or in-stent thrombosis.

In a subset of RAVEL, three-dimensional IVUS was used to characterize post-stent characteristics at 6 months [58]. Binary re-stenosis and late angiographic loss with the sirolimus stent was again eliminated at 6 months compared to the BMS (0% and 0.06 ± 0.30 mm versus 23.4% and 0.91 ± 0.58 mm) despite having a 21% incidence of incomplete stent apposition at 6 months compared to only 4% in the standard stent. While other trials have demonstrated

similar apposition rates using bare metal stents, the incomplete stent apposition compared to the control population is an intriguing finding that remains to be well explained [59, 60]. Perhaps there is a direct drug effect on local tissue that inhibits this apposition, however despite this finding, no patient with incomplete apposition in the sirolimus arm had an adverse event up to 1 year post procedure.

The SIRIUS trial then evaluated the Sirolimus stent compared to BMS in higher risk lesions [61]. Nine-month outcomes while not different in death or myocardial infarction demonstrated a marked reduction of target lesion revascularization (TLR) (4.1% versus 16.6%; $p < 0.001$), which continued out to 1 year. Characteristics associated with a high risk of restenosis were evaluated in the sub-group analysis [62] (Fig. 5.6). Twenty-six percent of patients (279 total) had diabetes mellitus. Both in-segment restenosis and TLR were markedly reduced, albeit higher than those without diabetes (Sirolimus stent: 17.6% and 6.9% versus BMS: 50.5% and 22.3%, respectively; $p < 0.001$). Additionally those with small vessels (2.29–2.32 mm) derived a significant benefit (TLR: 7.3% versus 20.6%; $p < 0.001$). In high risk lesions the sirolimus stent conferred a much improved event free survival mainly by reduced TLR compared to BMS.

Concurrently the Paclitaxel coated stent was being evaluated for its benefits in reducing restenosis. Paclitaxel, an immunomodulatory agent that stabilizes microtubules, thus arresting cells in the mitotic process, has also been shown to reduce vascular smooth muscle cell proliferation at local levels both in the animal and in vivo model [63–65]. The TAXUS I trial assessed the benefit of the eluting stent compared to BMS in single vessel lesions (length: <12 mm and diameters: 3.0–3.5 mm) [66]. In 61 patients, the major adverse cardiovascular event rates were less with the Paclitaxel stent compared to the bare metal stent (3% versus 10%; $p =$ NS) with no deaths or stent thrombosis. Additionally, 6-month IVUS evaluation revealed improved mean minimal lumen areas (5.6 mm^2 versus 4.8 mm^2, $p = 0.027$) as well as a reduction in neointimal hyperplasia (14.8 mm^3 versus 21.6 mm^3, $p = 0.028$). Despite a low risk subset, the Paclitaxel stent showed significant promise in the prevention of restenosis with a potential benefit in high risk lesions.

Variable	No. of Patients	Rate of Target-Lesion Revascularization (%)		Odds Ratio (95% CI)
		Sirolimus stent	Standard stent	
Overall	1058	4.1	16.6	
Male sex	753	4.4	16.6	
Female sex	305	3.4	16.5	
Diabetes				
Yes	279	6.9	22.3	
No	779	3.2	14.3	
Left anterior descending coronary artery				
Yes	462	5.1	19.8	
No	596	3.4	14.3	
Vessel diameter				
Small <2.75 mm	522	6.3	18.7	
Large ≥2.75 mm	523	1.9	14.8	
Lesion length				
≤13.5 mm	519	3.2	16.1	
>13.5 mm	519	5.2	17.4	
Overlapping stents				
Yes	344	4.5	17.7	
No	714	3.9	16.1	

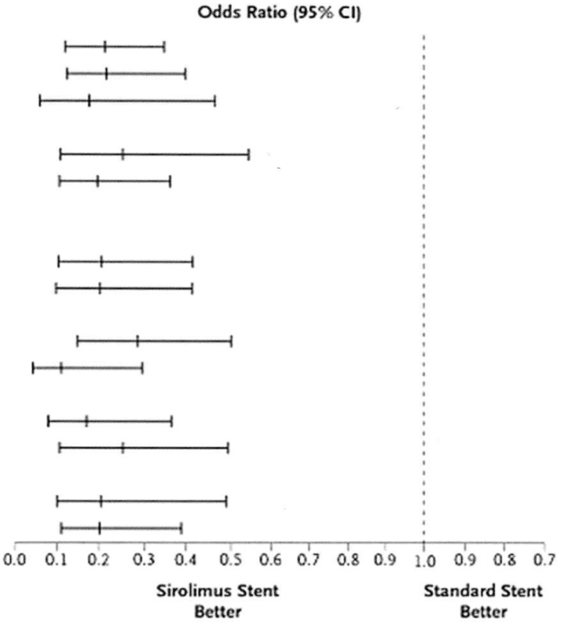

0.0 0.1 0.2 0.3 0.4 0.5 0.6 0.7 0.8 0.9 1.0 0.9 0.8 0.7

Sirolimus Stent Better   Standard Stent Better

Fig. 5.6 Sub-group analysis of SIRIUS drug eluting stent versus standard bare metal stenting at 270 days (© 2003, Massachusetts Medical Society)

The pivotal US trial for the Paclitaxel stent was the TAXUS IV trial, which enrolled 1,314 patients with single de novo coronary lesions (Length: 10–28 mm and diameter: 2.5–3.75 mm) [67] (Fig. 5.7). Target vessel revascularization based on ischemic symptoms was reduced from 12 to 4.7% ($p < 0.001$). The rate of restenosis by angiography was considerable lower (7.9% versus 26.6%; $p < 0.001$), with no difference in the rate of cardiac death, myocardial infarction, or stent thrombosis.

It now appears that drug-eluting stents have drastically reduced the rate of restenosis compared to the BMS counterparts; however, thus far no trial has proven superiority between the two commercially available drug-eluting stents. Current studies are ongoing to evaluate coated stents in high risk sub-sets including STEMI, decompensated heart failure, vein grafts, and high-risk lesions.

While drug eluting stents effectively tackled the problem of stent restenosis, other issues have emerged in recent times. In 2003, the FDA issued a warning regarding cases of sub-acute thrombosis (SAT) with the CYPHER stent that resulted in some deaths. This resulted in widespread media attention and concern among the patients. One potential explanation for the increased rate of SATs in Cypher-treated patients was that physicians were using the device "off-label" (i.e., for in-stent restenosis, long lesions, small vessels, etc.). However, it was also recognized that in most cases, DES were being used in cases where BMS was not suitable. Further study demonstrated that the rate of SAT was no higher among DES group than BMS group. In November 2003, the FDA recanted its earlier warning and confirmed the safety of the Cypher stent. One month later, the FDA also approved the second DES, TAXUS based on the TAXUS IV trial data. DES utilization continued to climb in the ensuing years.

In 2006, however, focus shifted to another rare but potentially catastrophic event known as "late stent thrombosis," which, in contrast to subacute thrombosis, occurs months to years after stent placement. It usually occurs before endothelialization is complete. For bare metal stents, this takes a few weeks. However, in drug eluting stents, this process of endotheliazation is delayed [68]. This complication

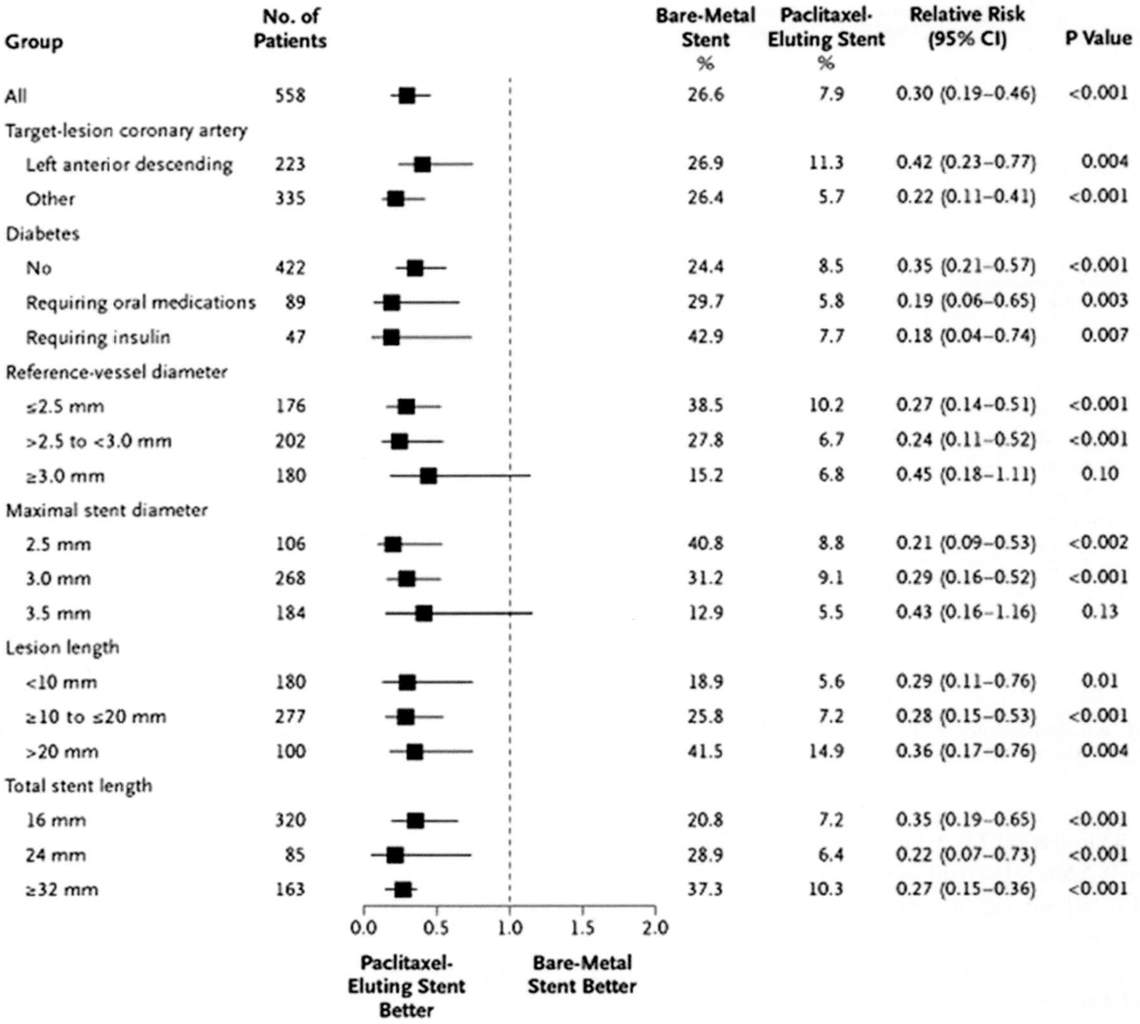

Group	No. of Patients		Bare-Metal Stent %	Paclitaxel-Eluting Stent %	Relative Risk (95% CI)	P Value
All	558		26.6	7.9	0.30 (0.19–0.46)	<0.001
Target-lesion coronary artery						
Left anterior descending	223		26.9	11.3	0.42 (0.23–0.77)	0.004
Other	335		26.4	5.7	0.22 (0.11–0.41)	<0.001
Diabetes						
No	422		24.4	8.5	0.35 (0.21–0.57)	<0.001
Requiring oral medications	89		29.7	5.8	0.19 (0.06–0.65)	0.003
Requiring insulin	47		42.9	7.7	0.18 (0.04–0.74)	0.007
Reference-vessel diameter						
≤2.5 mm	176		38.5	10.2	0.27 (0.14–0.51)	<0.001
>2.5 to <3.0 mm	202		27.8	6.7	0.24 (0.11–0.52)	<0.001
≥3.0 mm	180		15.2	6.8	0.45 (0.18–1.11)	0.10
Maximal stent diameter						
2.5 mm	106		40.8	8.8	0.21 (0.09–0.53)	<0.002
3.0 mm	268		31.2	9.1	0.29 (0.16–0.52)	<0.001
3.5 mm	184		12.9	5.5	0.43 (0.16–1.16)	0.13
Lesion length						
<10 mm	180		18.9	5.6	0.29 (0.11–0.76)	0.01
≥10 to ≤20 mm	277		25.8	7.2	0.28 (0.15–0.53)	<0.001
>20 mm	100		41.5	14.9	0.36 (0.17–0.76)	0.004
Total stent length						
16 mm	320		20.8	7.2	0.35 (0.19–0.65)	<0.001
24 mm	85		28.9	6.4	0.22 (0.07–0.73)	<0.001
≥32 mm	163		37.3	10.3	0.27 (0.15–0.36)	<0.001

0.0   0.5   1.0   1.5   2.0

Paclitaxel-Eluting Stent Better   Bare-Metal Stent Better

Fig. 5.7 TAXUS IV 9 month sub-group analysis of the Paclitaxel eluting stent versus comparative bare metal stent (© 2004 Massachusetts Medical Society)

had initially been reported in 2004 by Serruys et al. [69]. In 2006, three European studies presented at the World Congress of Cardiology suggested higher rates of late stent thrombosis than previously reported. A meta-analysis by Camenzind et al. of all available data from published randomized trials of Cypher (sirolimus-eluting stent) and Taxus (paclitaxel eluting stent) found a 38% higher relative risk of death or MI for Cypher patients than patients who received bare metal stents, and a 16% higher relative risk for patients implanted with Taxus stents versus those who received bare metal stents [70]. Data from the SCAAR registry from Sweeden showed increased

mortality in DES group starting at about 6 months after placement [71]. Over the following month, a slew of meta-analyses, subgroup analyses, registry reports emerged showing conflicting results. This received extensive media attention and contributed to the confusion. This forced the FDA to convene an advisory panel meeting to discuss stent thrombosis and the overall safety of DES [72]. The panel concluded that there appears to be a numerical excess of late stent thrombosis with DES, but the magnitude is uncertain. It was also recognized that a non-uniform definition of stent thrombosis and differences in study populations had contributed to apparently conflicting data [73]. They also noted that the off-label use of DES, as with BMS, is associated with increased risk when compared with on-label use. Nevertheless, DES use declined steeply worldwide.

Over the ensuing months, new criterion was proposed for defining stent-thrombosis in an attempt to establish uniformity, eliminate inappropriate censoring, and improve sensitivity.

Serruys et al. analyzed the patient level based data of the RAVEL, SIRUS, E-SIRIUS, and C-SIRIUS trails with a follow-up of 4 years using new standardized definitions of stent thrombosis and found that, in contrast to the data presented at ESC, the actual rate of total death and all MI at 4 years was not significantly different in the Cypher group (11.4%) vs the in the control group (10.1%) ($p = 0.4$) [74]. However, the time line of such events was different in the two groups. In DES, late ST occurs later than in BMS and seems to appear as primary thrombosis, whereas in BMS, a certain number of late thromboses are related to repeat interventions of the target lesion. Another study by Mauri et al. demonstrated that during 4 years of follow-up, overall rates of stent thrombosis were not significantly different for patients who had received either approved DES compared to those receiving BMS [75]. Stone et al. analyzed a pooled patient-level databse from four prospective trials of DES versus BMS and found that although DES may cause a small increase in the risk of late stent thrombosis resulting in death or MI, by markedly reducing the high rates of restenosis that would have occurred after BMS implantation, DES appeared to directly reduce the subsequent occurrence of death and non-fatal MI, offsetting the incremental stent thrombosis risk [76]. Updated results of the SCAAR registry data, presented at European Society of Cardiology Congress 2007, showed no overall increased risk of death for patients treated with DES as compared with bare-metal stents.

One of the significant factors promoting late stent thrombosis has been found to be premature discontinuation of dual antiplatelet therapy (aspirin and clopidrogel). In an analysis of 4,666 of patients undergoing initial PCI with BMS or DES, researchers from the Duke Heart center reported that long-term risk for death and major cardiac events was significantly increased among patients in the DES group who had discontinued clopidogrel therapy at 6 or 12 months. Specifically, among patients with DES who were event-free at 6 months, continued clopidogrel use was a significant predictor of lower adjusted rates of death (2.0% with versus 5.3% without; $p = 0.03$) and death or MI (3.1% versus 7.2%; $p = 0.02$) at 24 months [77]. As such, it has been stressed that dual Antiplatelet therapy be continued for at least 12 months after placement of a DES and premature discontinuation be avoided. It is also recommended that before implantation of a stent, the physician should discuss the need for dual antiplatelet therapy and in patients not expected to comply with 12 months of thienopyridine therapy, whether for economic or other reasons, strong consideration should be given to avoiding a DES [78].

The past 2 years have thus been a roller-coaster for drug eluting stents. However, one thing is clear. Preventing neointimal hyperplasia is no longer the ultimate goal [79]. Many new stent designs have been developed to reduce the rate of in-stent restenosis as well as late stent thrombosis. Bioabsorbable stents is one step in this direction. These stents are either polymer or metal based and designed to vanish away in a few months leaving behind only the healed natural vessel allowing restoration of vasoreactivity with the potential of vessel remodeling. This obviates the need for prolonged dual antiplatelet therapy without increasing the risk of late stent thrombosis. Preclinical studies of these stents showed no stent thrombosis and no significant differences in minimal lumen diameter at 6 months [80]. A magnesium based biocorridible stent was evaluated in the PROGRESS-AMS trial and showed no cases of stent thrombosis. However, the late lumen loss and TLR rates were high and comparable to bare metal stents. One-year follow-up of a Bioabsorbable Everolimus-Eluting Coronary Stent System (ABSORB trial) placed in a single de novo coronary artery lesion showed no cases of stent thrombosis demonstrated the feasibility and biocompatibility of bioabsorbable stents. However, the late lumen loss reported was higher than more than that with metallic everolimus-eluting stents. The late loss was mostly due to reduction in stent area from acute stent recoil, non-uniform structural support, or dwindling stent strength related to bioabsorption, but also because of intrastent neointimal hyperplasia [81]. Thus, more studies and more designs are needed to perfect this technology in the future.

Another avenue being explored is the development of newer anti-proliferative drugs. It is also hypothesized that the real culprit in stent thrombosis is the polymer and drug-release kinetics and not the stent itself [82]. Zotaralimus is a rapamycin analogue developed specifically for intravascular stents. The drug carrying polymer is phosphoryl-choline, a component of the lipid bilayer of the cell membrane and hence minimally thrombogenic and associated with rapid re-endothelialization and only mild inflammation in implanted coronary arteries [83]. Results from the ENDEAVOR IV trial, presented at TCT 2007, demonstrated non-inferiority of the Zotaralimus stent compared to paclitaxel eluting stent in the primary endpoint of target vessel failure. The ENDEAVOR stent was approved by the FDA in February 2008.

Another sirolimus analogue, Everolimus, on cobalt chromium stent platform (XIENCE V stent, Abbott Laboratories, Abbott Park, Illinois), was compared to the TAXUS stent in the SPIRIT III trial and found to have better MACE rates. The XIENCE V is approved in Europe and is awaiting FDA approval.

PCI in Patients with Left Ventricular Dysfunction

Patient with CAD and reduced left ventricular function are at a high risk of adverse events. From trials of CABG versus medical therapy, revascularization provided a significant mortality benefit; however, in higher risk sub-groups there remained an early increase in morbidity [84–87]. In the CASS study, the survival benefit at 7 years was 84 versus 70% ($p = 0.01$) in patients with moderately reduced LVEF (>35 but <50%), which is more dramatic in those patients with triple vessel disease (88% versus 65%; $p < 0.009$). These trials enrolled symptomatic patients, with limited data on the benefits of revascularization in those with silent ischemia. Tillisch et al. found that those with significant wall motion abnormalities are more likely to improve from CABG, and viability scanning with SPECT, PET, or Dobutamine stress echo can further improve revascularization strategies [88, 89]. In a meta-analysis of 24 studies of ischemic cardiomyopathy, revascularization in patients with viability was associated with a profound reduction in mortality compared to those with viable myocardium and no revascularization (3.2% versus 16%; $p < 0.001$) [90]. Benefits of revascularization and severity of LV dysfunction were significantly related; however, those patients without viability had no benefit of revascularization despite their level of ventricular dysfunction.

The more recent use of aggressive medical therapy with beta blockers, ACE-inhibitors, aspirin, and HMG CoA reductase inhibitors has had a profound benefit on those with coronary artery disease and reduced LVEF. To that end, revascularization still plays an important role in mortality reduction. In the Studies of Left Ventricular Dysfunction (SOLVD) database, CABG does improve survival compared to more modern use of medical therapy, with a 25% mortality risk reduction as well as an intriguing 46% risk reduction of sudden death [91]. This benefit improved as LVEF decreased, thus providing evidence that revascularization may stabilize heart function, reduce abnormal remodeling, and thus reduce the propensity to arrhythmogenicity.

Few studies have been completed to evaluate the use of PCI in this unique population. Early studies of PTCA showed promise with a 1- and 4-year survival in patients with LVEF <40% being 86% and 69%, respectively, with 59% of patients angina free (mean follow-up 33.5 months) [92]. The NHLBI PTCA registry evaluated the risk of depressed LVEF on outcomes. Those with LVEF <45% compared to normal LVEF were more likely to have multivessel disease, prior infarction, history of coronary artery bypass surgery, as well as total occlusions. Due to higher lesion risk, there was a decreased incidence of complete revascularization (35% versus 47%; $p < 0.001$) as well as successful dilatation (76% versus 84%; $p < 0.01$). In-hospital complications including death were similar between both groups; however, not surprisingly, those with impaired function had comparatively poor long term outcomes (4-year mortality and freedom from myocardial infarction: 23% versus 17%; $p < 0.05$). Five-year review of the registry revealed that CHF increased the risk of mortality from both cardiac and non-cardiac causes [93]. With this data, revascularization could have a profound benefit and PCI with lower early morbidity compared to CABG could be a viable option.

With the advent of PCI, interventionalists are undertaking higher risk lesions including those with depressed LVEF. Despite further advances, there remains a significant association between LVEF and 1-year mortality compared to normal systolic function. More interesting is the comparison of revascularization strategies. Toda et al. compared CABG versus PCI in those patients with severe dysfunction (LVEF: 15–30%) [94]. While those undergoing CABG were more likely to have complete revascularization 3-year mortality was no different between the two strategies (73% versus 67%). The elderly and those without proximal LAD stenosis had similar rates of cardiac events as well as target vessel revascularization. While there would be a theoretical benefit to complete revascularization, this demonstrated that even in those patients with low ejection fraction, PCI could stabilize systolic function with similar midterm survival to complete therapy. To date there is no data to evaluate the benefits of drug eluting stent technology in this population. Currently on going are large registry databases as well as TAXUS V and VI, which aim to address this unique sub-set.

Conclusion

Percutaneous coronary intervention has come a long way from the days of our founding interventional fathers. Improvements in medical therapy and the increasing breath of knowledge regarding the pathophysiologic, genetic, and molecular basis for CHF has improved our current treatment modalities. PCI is a viable option for those with advanced ischemic disease and with the advent of drug eluting stent technology, the risk of repeat procedures is drastically minimized. We must closely evaluate the role of the interventionalist in CHF therapy as well as the benefits of complete revascularization. Further advances in stent design and support devices will allow treatment of higher risk lesions with a high procedural success and limited adverse outcomes.

References

1. Nobel Lecture, Physics, 1901–1921, Elsevier Publishing Company, Amsterdam, 1967.
2. Cournand AF, Riley RL, Breed ES, et al. Measurement of cardiac output in man using the technique of catheterization of the right auricle. J Clin Invest 1945;24:106.
3. Richard DW. Cardiac output in the catherization technique in various clinical conditions. Fed Proc 1945;4:215.
4. Nobel Lectures, Physiology or Medicine 1942–1962, Elsevier Publishing Company, Amsterdam, 1964.
5. Sones FM. Cine coronary angiography. Mod Concepts Cardiovasc Dis 1962;31:735–738.
6. Dotter C, Judkins MP. Transluminal treatment of arteriosclrotic obstruction: description of a new technique and preliminary report on its application. Circulation 1964;30:654.
7. Dotter CT, Rosch J, Anderson JM, et al. Transluninal iliac artery dilatation: nonsurgical catheter treatment of atheromatous narrowing. JAMA 1978;230:117.
8. Dotter CT. Transluminal angioplasty: a long view. Radiology 1980;135:561.
9. Favalaro RG. Saphenous vein graft in the surgical treatment of coronary artery disease: operative technique. J Thorac Cariovasc Surg 1969;58:178.
10. Greuntzig AR, Turina MI, Schneider JA. Experimental percutaneous dilatation of coronary artery stenosis. Circulation 1976;54:81.
11. Greuntzig AR. Translumination dilatation of coronary artery stenosis. Lancet 1978;1:263.
12. Simpson JB, Baim DS, Robert EW, Harrison DC. A new catheter system for coronary angioplasty. Am J Cardiol 1982;49:1216.
13. Detre K, Peduzzi P, Murphy M, et al. Effect of bypass surgery on survival in patients with low and high risk subgroups delineated by use of simple clinical variable. Circulation 1981;63:1329.
14. Murphy ML, Hultgren HN, Detre K, et al. Treatment of chronis stable angina: a preliminary report of survival data of the randomized Veterans Administration Cooperative Study. N Engl J Med 1977;297:621.
15. CASS Principal Investigators and their Associates. Myocardial infarction and mortality in the Coronary Artery Surgery Study. N Engl J Med 1984;310:750.
16. Yusuf S, Zucker D, Peduzzi P, et al. Effect of coronary artery bypass surgery on survival: overview of 10 year results from randomized rials by the Coronary Artery Bypass Surgery Trialists Collaboration. Lancet 1994;344:563.
17. Parisi AF, Folland ED, Hertigan P. A comparison of angioplasty with medical therapy in the treatment of single-vessel coronary artery disease. N Engl J Med 1992;326:10.
18. Folland ED, Hartigan PM, Parisi AF. Percutaneous transluminal coronary angioplasty versus medical therapy for stable angina pectoris: outcomes for patients with double-vessel versus single—vessel coronary artery disease in a Vererans Affairs cooperative randomized trial. J Am Coll Cardiol 1997;29:1505.

19. RITA 2 Trial Participants. Coronary angioplasty versus medical therapy for angina; The second Randomized Intervention Treatment of Angina trial. Lancer 1997;350:461.
20. Hueb WA Bellotti G, de Oliveira SA, et al. The Medicine, Angioplasty and Surgery Study: a prospective, randomized trial of medical therapy, balloon angioplasty, or bypass surgery for single proximal left anterior descending artery stenosis. J Am Coll Cardiol 1995;26:606.
21. RITA Trial Participants. Coronary angioplasty vs. coronary artery bypass surgery: the randomized intervention treatment of angina trial. Lancet 1993;341:573.
22. Rodriguez A, Boullon F, Perez-Balino N, et al. Argentine randomized trial of percutaneous transluminal coronary angioplasty versus coronary artery bypass surgery in multivessel disease: in-hospital results and 1 year follow-up. J Am Coll Cardiol 1993;22:1060.
23. Rogers WJ, Alderman EL, Chaitman BR, et al. Bypass angioplasty revasculariztion investigation: baseline clinical and angiographic data. Am J Cardiol 1995;75:9C.
24. Waller BF. "Crackers, breakers, stretchers, drillers, scrapers, shavers, burners, welders and melters"—the future treatment of atherosclerotic coronary artery disease? a clinical-morphologic assessment. J Am Coll Cardiol 1989;13:969–987.
25. Serruys PW, de Jaegere P, Kiemeneij F, et al., for the BENESTENT study group. A comparison of balloon-expandable stent implantation with balloon angioplasty in patients with coronary artery disease. N Engl J Med 1994;331:489–495.
26. Fischman DL, Leon MB, Baim DS, et al., for the Stent Restenosis Study Investigators. A randomized comparison of coronary stent placement and balloon angioplasty in the treatment of coronary artery disease. N Engl J Med 1994;331:496–501.
27. Serruys PW, Unger F, Sousa JE, et al. Comparison of coronary bypass surgery and stenting for the treatment of multivesel disease. N Engl J Med 2001;344:1117–1124.
28. Serruys P, Ong A, van Herwerden L, et al. Five-year outcomes after coronary stenting versus bypass surgery for the treatment of multivessel disease. J Am Coll Cardiol 2005; 46:575–581.
29. Rodriguez A, Bernardi V, Navia J, et al. Argentine randomized study: coronary angioplasty wih stenting versus coronary artery bypass surgery in patients with multiple vessel disease: 30-day and one year follow-up results. J Am Coll Cardiol 2001;37:51–58.
30. Rodriguez A, Baldi J, Pereira C, et al. Five-year follow-up of the argentine randomized trial of coronary angioplasty with stenting versus coronary bypass surgery in patients with multiple vessel disease. J Am Coll Cardiol 2005;46:583–588.
31. Effects of tissue plasminogen activator and a comparison of early invasive and conservative strategies in unstable angina and non-Q-wave myocardial infarction: results of the TIMI IIIB trial. Thrombolysis in myocardial ischemia. Circulation 1994;89:1545–1556.
32. Baigent C, Collins R, Appleby P, Parish S, Sleight P, Peto R, for the ISIS-2 (Second International Study of Infarct Survival) Collaborative Group. ISIS-2: 10 year

survival among patients with suspected acute myocardial infarction in randomised comparison of intravenous streptokinase, oral aspirin, both, or neither. BMJ 1998;316:1337–1343.
33. Franzosi MG, Santoro E, De Vita C, et al. Ten-year follow-up of the first megatrial testing thrombolytic therapy in patients with acute myocardial infarction: results of the Gruppo Italiano per lo Studio della Sopravvivenza nell'Infarto-1 study. The GISSI Investigators. Circulation 1998;98:2659–2665.
34. TIMI IIIB Investigators. Effects of tissue plasminogen activator and a comparison of early invasive and conservative strategies in unstable angina and non-Q wave myocardial infarction. Circulation 1994;89:1545.
35. Wallentin L, Lagerqvist B, Husted S, et al. Outcome at 1-year after an invasive compared with a non-invasive strategy in unstable coronary artery disease (FRISC-2). Lancet 2000;359:9–16.
36. Boden WE, O'Rourke RA, Crawford MH, et al. Outcomes in patients with acute non-Q wave myocardial infarction randomly assigned to an invasive as compared with a conservative management strategy (VANQUISH). N Engl J Med 1998;338:1785–1792.
37. Cannon C, Weintraub W, Demopoulos L, et al. Comparison of early invasive and conservative strategies in patients with unstable coronary syndromes treated with Glycoprotein IIb/IIIa inhibitor Tirofiban. N Engl J of Med 2001;344:1879–1887.
38. Gruppo Italiano per lo Studio della Streptochinasi nell'Infarto Miocardico (GISSI): Effectiveness of intravenous thrombolytic treatment in acute myocardial infarction. Lancet 1986;1:397–402.
39. ISIS-2 (Second International Study of Infarct Survival) Collaborative Group. Randomized trial of intravenous streptokinase, oral aspirin, both, or neither among 17,187 cases of suspected acute myocardial infarction: ISIS-2. Lancet 1988;2:349–360.
40. Meijer A, Verheugt FW, Werter CJ, Lie KI, van der Pol JM, van Eenige MJ. Aspirin versus coumadin in the prevention of reocclusion and recurrent ischemia after successful thrombolysis: a prospective placebo-controlled angiographic study. Results of the APRICOT Study. Circulation 1993;87:1524–1530.
41. O'Keefe JH, Jr., Rutherford BD, McConahay DR, et al. Early and late results of coronary angioplasty without antecedent thrombolytic therapy for acute myocardial infarction. Am J Cardiol 1989;64: 1221–1230.
42. Rothbaum DA, Linnemeier TJ, Landin RJ, et al. Emergency percutaneous transluminal coronary angioplasty in acute myocardial infarction: a 3 year experience. J Am Coll Cardiol 1987;10:264–272.
43. Grines CL, Browne KF, Oneil W, et al., for the Primary Angioplasty in Myocardial Infarction study group. A comparison of immediate angioplasty with thrombolytic therapy for acute myocardial infarction. N Engl J Med 1993;328:673–679.
44. Zijlstra F, de Boer M, Hoorntje J, et al. Comparison of immediate coronary angioplasty with intravenous streptokinase in myocardial infarction. N Eng J Med 1993;328:680–684.

45. Cannon CP, Gibson CM, Lambrew CT. Relationship of symptom onset to balloon time and door to balloon time with the mortality in patients undergoing angioplasty for acute myocardial infarction. JAMA 2000;283:2941–2947.
46. Nagakawa Y, Iwasaki Y, Kimura T, et al. Serial angiographic follow-up after successful direct angioplasty for acute myocardial infarction. Am J Cardiol 1996;78:980–984.
47. Grines CL, Cox DA, Stone GW, et al. Coronary angioplasty with or without stent implantation for acute myocardial infarction. N Engl J Med 1999;341:1949–1956.
48. Maillard L, Hamon M, Khalife K, et al. A comparison of systematic stenting and conventional balloon angioplasty during primary percutaneous transluminal coronary angioplasty for acute myocardial infarction. J Am Coll Cardiol 2000;35:1729–1736.
49. Antoniucci D, Santoro GM, Bolognese L, et al. A clinical trial comparing primary stenting of the infarct related artery with optimal primary angioplasty for acute myocardial infarction (FRESCO). J Am Coll Cardiol 1998;31:1234–1239.
50. Lefkovits J, Ivanhoe RJ, Califf RM, et al. Effects of platelet glycoprotein IIb/IIIa receptor blockade by a chimeric monoclonal antibody on acute and six-month outcomes after percutaneous transluminal coronary angioplasty for acute myocardial infarction (EPIC). Am J Cardiol 1996;77:1045–1051.
51. Antman E, et al. ACC/AHA guidelines for the management of patients with ST-elevation myocardial infarction-Executive summary. J Am Coll Cardiol 2004;44:671–719.
52. Cutlip DE, Chauhan MS, Baim DS, et al. Clinical restenosis after coronary stenting: perspectives from multicenter trials. J Am Coll Cardiol 2002;40:2082–2089.
53. Hausleiter J, Kastrati A, Mehili J, et al. Predictive factors for early cardiovascular events and angiographic restenosis after coronary stent placement in small coronary arteries. J Am Coll Cardiol 2002;40:882–889.
54. Kereiakes D, Linnemeier TJ, Baim DS, et al. Usefulness of stent length in predicting in-stent restenosis (the MULTI-LINK stent trials). Am J Cardiol 2000;86:336–341.
55. Marx SO, Jayaraman T, Go LO, et al. Rapamycin-FKBP inhibits cell cycle regulators of proliferation in vascular smooth muscle cells. Circ Res 1995;76:412–417.
56. Poon M, Marx SO, Gallo R, et al. Rapamycin inhibits vascular smooth muscle cell migration. J Clin Invest 1996;98:2277–2283.
57. Morice MC, Serruys PW, Sousa E, et al. A randomized comparison of a sirolimus-eluting stent with a standard stent for coronary revascularization. NEJM 2002;346:1773–1780.
58. Surruys PW, Degertekin M, Tanabe K, et al. Intravascular ultrasound findings in the multicenter randomized, double-blind RAVEL trial. Circulation 2002;106:798–803.
59. Kobayashi Y, Honda Y, Christie LG, et al. Long-term vessel response to a self-expanding coronary stent: a serial volumetric intravascular ultrasound analysis from the ASSURE trial. J Am Coll Cardiol 2001; 1329–1334.
60. Uren NG, Schwarzacher SP, Metz JA, et al. Predictors and outcomes of stent thrombosis: an intrazvascular ultrasound registry. Eur Heart J 2002;23:124–132.
61. Holmes DR Jr, Leon MB, Moses JW, Popma JJ, Cutlip D, Fitzgerald PJ, Brown C, Fischell T, Wong SC, Midei M, Snead D, Kuntz RE. Analysis of 1-year clinical outcomes in the SIRIUS trial: a randomized trial of a sirolimus-eluting stent versus a standard stent in patients at high risk for coronary restenosis. Circulation. 2004 Feb 10;109(5):634–40.
62. Moses J, Leon M, Popma J, et al. Sirolimus-eluting stents versus standard stents in patients with stenosis in a native coronary artery. N Engl J Med 2003;349:1315–1323.
63. Axel DI, Kunert W, Goggelmann C, et al. Paclitaxel inhibits arterial smooth muscle cell proliferation and migration in vitro and in vivo using local drug delivery. Circulation 1997;96:636–645.
64. Hanke H, Oberhoff M, Hanke S, Hassenstein S, Kamenz J, Schmid KM, Betz E, Karsch KR. Inhibition of cellular proliferation after experimental balloon angioplasty by low-molecular-weight heparin. Circulation 1992;85:1548–1556.
65. Schwartz RS, Holmes DR, Topol EJ. The restenosis paradigm revisited: an alternative proposal for cellular mechanisms. J Am Coll Cardiol 1992;20: 1284–1293.
66. Grube E, Silber S, Hauptmann KE, et al. Six and twelve-month results from a randomized, double blind tial on a slow-release Paclitaxel-eluting stent for de novo coronary lesion. Circulation 2003;107:38–42.
67. Stone G, Ellis S, Cox D, et al. A polymer-based, Paclitaxel-eluting stent in patients with coronary artery disease. N Eng J Med 2004;350:221–231.
68. Joner M, Finn AV, Farb A, et al. Pathology of drug-eluting stents in humans: delayed healing and late thrombotic risk. J Am Coll Cardiol 2006;48:193–202.
69. McFadden EP, Stabile E, Regar E, et al. Late thrombosis in drug-eluting coronary stents after discontinuation of antiplatelet therapy. Lancet 2004;364:1519–1521.
70. Camenzind E. Do drug-eluting stent increase death? ESC Congress News. Barcelona, Spain; 2006.
71. Lagerqvist B, James SK, Stenestrand U, Lindbäck J, Nilsson T, Wallentin L, SCAAR Study Group. Long-term outcomes with drug-eluting stents versus bare-metal stents in Sweden. N Engl J Med 2007 Mar 8;356(10):1009–1019
72. US Food and Drug Administration. Circulatory System Devices Panel. Available at http://www.fda.gov/ohrms/dockets/ac/cdrh06.html#circulatory
73. William HM. Unanswered questions—drug-eluting stents and the risk of late thrombosis. N Engl J Med 2007 Mar 8;356(10):981–984.
74. Serruys PW, Daemen J. Are drug-eluting stents associated with a higher rate of late thrombosis than bare metal stents? Late stent thrombosis: a nuisance in both bare metal and drug-eluting stents. Circulation 2007;115:1433–1439.
75. Mauri L, Hsieh WH, Massaro JM, et al. Stent thrombosis in randomized clinical trials of drug-eluting stents. N Engl J Med 2007;356:1020–1029.

76. Stone GW, Ellis SG, Colombo A, Dawkins KD, Grube E, Cutlip DE, Friedman M, Baim DS, Koglin J. Offsetting impact of thrombosis and restenosis on the occurrence of death and myocardial infarction after paclitaxel-eluting and bare metal stent implantation. Circulation 2007 Jun 5;115(22):2842–2847.

77. Eisenstein EL, Anstrom KJ, Kong DF, et al. Clopidogrel use and long-term clinical outcomes after drug-eluting stent implantation. JAMA 2007;297:159–168.

78. Grines CL, Bonow RO, Casey DE, et al. Prevention of premature discontinuation of dual antiplatelet therapy in patients with coronary artery stents: a science advisory. J Am Coll Cardiol 2007;49:734–739.

79. Serruys PW, Daemen J. Are drug-eluting stents associated with a higher rate of late thrombosis than bare metal stents? Late stent thrombosis: a nuisance in both bare metal and drug-eluting stents. Circulation 2007;115:1433–1439.

80. Tamai H, Igaki K, Tsuji T, et al. A biodegradable poly-L-lactic acid coronary stent in porcine coronary artery. J Interv Cardiol 1999;12:443–450.

81. Ormiston J, Serruys PW, Regar E, et al. A bioabsorbable everolimus-eluting coronary stent system for patients with single de-novo coronary artery lesions (ABSORB): a prospective open-label trial. *Lancet* 2008;371:899–907.

82. Kornowski R, Hong MK, Tio FO, Bramwell O, Wu H, Leon MB. In-stent restenosis: contributions of inflammatory responses and arterial injury to neointimal hyperplasia. J Am Coll Cardiol 1998;31:224–230.

83. Whelan DM, van der Giessen WJ, Krabbendam SC, van Vliet EA, Verdouw PD, Serruys PW, van Beusekom HM. Biocompatibility of phosphorylcholine coated stents in normal porcine coronary arteries. Heart 2000;83:338–345.

84. Passamani E, Davis KB, Gillespie MJ, et al. A randomized trial of coronary artery bypass surgery: Survival of patients with a low ejection fraction. N Engl J Med 1985;312:1665–1671.

85. Scott SM, Luchi RJ, Deupree RH, et al. Veterans Administration cooperative srudy for the treatment of patients with unstable angina: Results in patients with abnormal left ventricular function. Circulation 1988;78(suppl I):I-113–I-121.

86. Naunheim KS, Fiore AC, Wadley JJ, et al. The changing profile of the patient undergoing coronary artery bypass surgery. J Am Coll Cardiol 1988;11:494–498.

87. Kennedy JW, Kaiser GC, Fisher LD, et al. Multivariate discriminant analysis of the clinical and angiographic predictors of operative mortality form the collaborative study in coronary artery surgery (CASS). J Thorac Cardiovasc Surg 1980;80:876–887.

88. Luu M, Stevenson LW, Brunken RC, et al. Delayed recovery of revascularized myocardium after referral for cardiac transplantation. Am Heart J 1990;119:668–670.

89. Tillisch J, Brunken R, Marshall R, et al. Reversibility of cardiac wall motion abnormalities predicted by positron tomography. N Engl J Med 1986;314: 884–888.

90. Allman KC, Shaw LJ, Hachamovitch R, Udelson J. Myocardial viability testing and impact of revascularization on prognosis in patients with coronary artery disease and left ventricular dysfunction: a meta analysis. J Am Coll Cardiol 2002;39:1151–1158.

91. Veenhuyzen GD, Sing SN, McAreavey D, et al. Prior coronary artery bypass surgery and risk of death among patients with ischemic left ventricular dysfunction. Circulation 2001;104:1489–1493.

92. Stevens T, Kahn JK, McCallister BD, et al. Safety and efficacy of percutaneous transluminal coronary angioplasty in patients with left ventricular dysfunction. Am J Cardiol 1991;68:313–319.

93. Holmes DR, Kip KE, Kelsey SF, et al. Cause of death analysis in the NHLBI PTCA registry: results and considerations for evaluating long-term survival after coronary interventions. J Am Coll Cardiol 1997;30:881–887.

94. Toda K, Mackenzie K, Mehra MR, DiCorte CJ, Davis JE, McFadden PM, Ochsner JL, White C, Van Meter CH Jr;. Revascularization in severe ventricular dysfunction (15% < OR = LVEF < OR = 30%): a comparison of bypass grafting and percutaneous intervention. Ann Thorac Surg. 2002 Dec;74(6):2082–7.

Chapter 6
Percutaneous Mechanical Assist Devices

Currently Available Devices, Their Indications and Usages, Patient Selection and Management

Harvinder Singh Arora and Reynolds Delgado

Introduction

Although impressive developments have taken place in the pharmacologic treatment of heart failure, most of these treatments have failed to improve the prognosis in stage D heart failure [1]. While heart transplantation remains the most established treatment for refractory heart failure, shortage of donor hearts [2] has necessitated development of alternative forms of therapy. Mechanical support devices have been used for the past few decades in advanced heart failure either as a bridge to transplantation or as destination therapy. The majority of these devices consist of mechanical pumps that need surgery for implantation and explantation. Surgery in this critically sick population is associated with a high morbidity and mortality risk. Also, the size of most of these devices precludes a significant percentage of patients from receiving the benefit of mechanical circulatory support.

Over the years, focus has shifted to developing pumps that can be deployed in the catheterization laboratory. Percutaneous LVADs have been developed for rapid deployment in the catheterization laboratory to provide short-term hemodynamic support without the risks of major surgery. The spectrum of percutaneous circulatory support therapy ranges from the intra-aortic balloon pump (IABP), which reduces cardiac work by reducing afterload and increases coronary perfusion, to the current generation of pumps that offer more effective myocardial unloading to allow for greater support and recovery of function.

Intra Aortic Balloon Counterpulsation

Since Kantrovitz et al. described the concept of counterpulsation in 1968 [3], the IABP has been the mainstay for temporarily augmenting the cardiac output and improving hemodynamics in acutely decompensated refractory HF [4, 5]. IABP use has been shown to reduce heart rate, left ventricular end-diastolic pressure, mean left atrial pressure, afterload, and myocardial oxygen consumption by at least 20–30%. The IABP also modestly increases coronary perfusion pressure and decreases the right atrial pressure, pulmonary artery pressure, and pulmonary vascular resistance [6].

The pump's major advantages are its ease of use and wide availability. Frequent IABP use is speculated to have been a factor affecting the low 30-day mortality of the medically treated group in the SHOCK (Should we emergently revascularize Occluded Coronaries for cardiogenic shocK?) trial [7]. However, other studies suggest that the IABP only delays death and does not prevent it [8]. The IABP's main limitations are its short duration of use and requirement for partially intact left ventricular function [9].

H.S. Arora (✉)
Texas Heart Institute, St. Luke's Episcopal Hospital,
Houston, TX, USA
e-mail: harora@bcm.tmc.edu

R. Delgado, H.S. Arora (eds.), *Interventional Treatment of Advanced Ischemic Heart Disease*,
DOI 10.1007/978-1-84800-395-8_6, © Springer-Verlag London Limited 2009

Rationale for Ventricular Support Therapy

Cardiogenic shock, whether due to acute heart failure, ischemic cardiomyopathy (ICM), or non-ischemic cardiomyopathy (NICM) is associated with high mortality despite adequate medical therapy. In the SHOCK trial, about two thirds of the patients died in the medically treated group [7]. Inotropes acutely increases cardiac output, but at a cost of increased myocardial work, oxygen demand, and an increased arrhythmia risk. There is good evidence that prolonged inotrope use actually worsens prognosis [10, 11].

Mechanical support, on the other hand, combines the beneficial effects of myocardial unloading and maintenance of end-organ perfusion. Unloading of the myocardium leads to functional, structural, signaling, and molecular changes in the myocardium [12]. Observations on isolated myocytes have shown recovery of contractile function and ß-adrenergic responsiveness [13], as well as regression in cellular hypertrophy [14, 15] and fibrosis after prolonged mechanical support. Echocardiographic studies have also demonstrated a decrease in end diastolic dimensions and left ventricular mass [16]. An important observation in studies with surgically placed mechanical assist devices was the phenomenon of profound cardiac recovery in some patients supported with devices who were thought to have irreversible HF [17]. In a recent study, a combination of mechanical unloading and pharmacological therapy was used to produce substantial functional improvement that allowed explantation of the device without the need of transplantation in patients with dilated cardiomyopathy [18].

The initial generation of mechanical pumps was used to stabilize patients until a donor heart becomes available. In 2001, the REMATCH trial demonstrated the use of LVADs as "destination therapy" in patients with heart failure ineligible for transplantation [19]. In a minority of patients, the pumps are used as "bridge to recovery" [17].

Mechanical support therapy has been a significant addition to the armamentarium against refractory heart failure. However, surgically placed pumps are associated with significant morbidity and mortality, most related to the surgical implantation procedure itself [19]. Because of the limits of surgical implantation, alternative pumps have been developed that can be rapidly deployed in the catheterization lab, without exposing an already frail patient to the risk of major surgery [20].

The currently available percutaneously implanted pumps offer short term ventricular support only. They have been mostly used in acute cardiogenic shock to provide acute hemodynamic stability before another definitive therapy like revascularization, surgical LVAD, or transplantation. Following is a description of the currently available percutaneous LVADs.

TandemHeart

The TandemHeart (Cardiac Assist, Inc., Pittsburgh, PA) (Fig. 6.1) is an extracorporeal, continuous flow, centrifugal pump used for brief support (up to 3 weeks). It can be implanted in the catheterization laboratory or in the operating room. The device consists of a 21 French inlet cannula, which is placed in the femoral vein and fed up through the inferior vena cava into the right atrium across the septum and sits in the left atrium. The tip of the cannula has nine holes to drain the blood from the left atrium to the inflow of the pump. Oxygenated blood is withdrawn from the left atrium through this inlet cannula into an external electrical impeller which then propels the blood, through the outflow cannula (15–17 F), into the femoral artery. The external pump is a low prime volume (<10 cc) centrifugal pump driven by a three phase, brushless, DC servomotor capable of delivering 5 l/min of blood flow at 7,500 rpm (rotations per minute). Instead of conventional mechanical roller bearings, this design uses a hydrodynamic fluid bearing that supports the spinning rotor. The fluid bearing is supplied by a unique lubrication system that feeds a nominal 10 cc/h of saline to which an anticoagulant (usually Heparin) is added. The fluid acts as a coolant and lubricant for the seal that separates the rotor chamber from the blood chamber. An external microprocessor-based controller regulates the impeller speed and lubricant flow with automatic system monitoring and alarms. Because

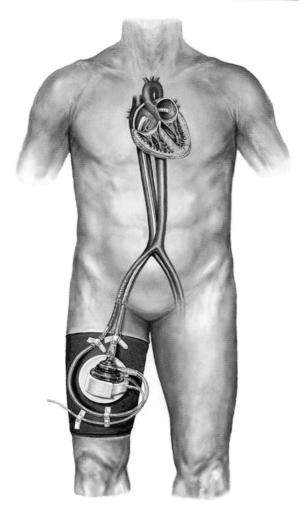

Fig. 6.1 TandemHeart consists of an extracorporeal pump, an inlet cannula in the left atrium, and an outlet cannula in the femoral artery

explantation of the transseptal cannula, which resolves after 4–6 weeks and is usually of no clinical consequence [19].

In patients with cardiogenic shock, the Tandem-Heart has been shown to significantly reduce PCWP, ventricular workload, and myocardial oxygen demand and increase cardiac output and mean arterial pressure even in patients refractory to the IABP, although no survival benefit has been observed [21]. In this study, there was also a significantly increased incidence of limb ischemia, bleeding, DIC, and need for PLT transfusions with Tandem-Heart compared to IABP. Other reported complications include stroke, infection, arterial/venous laceration/dissection, atrial/pulmonary vein perforation, air embolism, right ventricular failure, ARDS, and PFO with right to left shunting. Table 6.1 describes the effect of TandemHeart on various hemodynamic and clinical parameters in our experience at the Texas Heart Institute.

Although an effective device, widespread utilization is limited by the need for trans-septal cannulation. Severe peripheral vascular disease is a contraindication for TandemHeart, an often present co-morbid condition. Optimal pump performance is dependent on adequate filling pressures. Any condition that leads to a decrease in left atrial filling will affect pump flow. Possible causes are as follows: right sided circulatory failure pulmonary hypertension, bleeding, hypovolemia, tamponade, and arrhythmias.

In July 2003, TandemHeart received 510(k) approval from the FDA for short-term (up to 6 h) use in refractory cardiogenic shock. Subsequently, the duration of use was extended up to 3 weeks. It is also being evaluated as a bridge to long-term ventricular assistance and as a means of cardiac support in high-risk interventional procedures [22].

of the size of inlet and outlet cannulas, explantation requires surgical repairs of vessels. A small iatrogenic atrial septal defect is left after the

Table 6.1 Effect of TandemHeart use on various parameters in refractory cardiogenic shock—Texas Heart Institute experience

	Pre TandemHeart	Post TandemHeart	*P* value
CI (lpm)	0.7 ± 0.5	2.79 ± 0.97	<0.0001
SVO2 (%)	39 ± 10	66 ± 8	<0.0001
PCWP (mmHg)	29 ± 9	14 ± 5	<0.0001
SBP (mmHg)	79 ± 20	101 ± 13	<0.0001
Lactic acid (mg/dl)	64 ± 54	27 ± 30	<0.03
Creatinine (mg/dl)	2.3 ± 1.3	1.5 ± 0.7	<0.02

Current and Future Indications for Percutaneous Support Devices

1. Cardiogenic Shock
2. High risk coronary intervention, high risk PCI
3. Large AMI involving 30% or more of anterior wall
4. Valve surgery with severe aortic stenosis or mitral regurgitation
5. Ruptured papillary muscle or VSD
6. Ventricular tachycardia and high risk bi-ventricular pacing
7. Acute decompensated heart failure, myocarditis, or severe myopathy
8. Systolic pressure <80 mmHg after revascularization
9. Isolated right heart failure as RVAD

Impella Recovery System

The Impella Recovery System (Abiomed, Inc., Danvers, MA) (Fig. 6.2A and B) consists of an miniature axial flow impeller mounted on a 12 French catheter, with a suction chamber in the left ventricle and an outlet in the ascending aorta. The Impella pump has both percuatneous and surgical variants. The Impella Recover 2.5 is inserted retrogradely over a 0.014 in. wire through a 13 F peel away sheath in the femoral artery. High speed rotation of the microaxial impeller aspirates blood through the blood inlet positioned in the LV, from where it is directed through a hollow nitinol tube and ejected past the impeller into the ascending aorta. There is a pressure sensor at the tip of the catheter that monitors pressure difference between the left ventricle and the ascending aorta. Up to 2.5 l of blood per minute are delivered by the pump from the left ventricle into the ascending aorta [20]. The Impella® LP5.0 can deliver up to 5 l/min but needs a small cut-down of the femoral artery.

Animal studies with the Impella pump have demonstrated a decrease in myocardial oxygen demand during ischemia and reperfusion, resulting in a smaller infarct size [23]. Initial experience in patients with cardiogenic shock treated with the Impella pump system showed improvements in cardiac output and mean blood pressure and a reduction in pulmonary capillary wedge pressure [24].

(A)
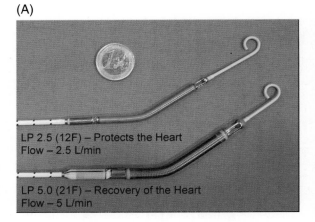

(B)
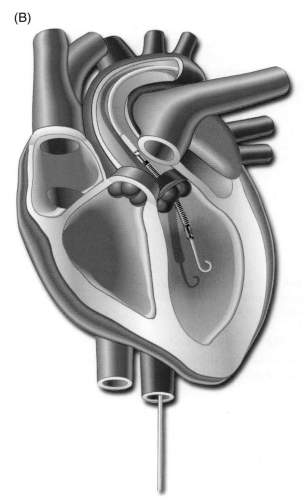

Fig. 6.2 (**A**) The Impella pump is a miniature flow mounted pump. It comes in two different sizes and can produce cardiac output of 2.5–5 l/min. (**B**) The Impella pump is placed across the aortic valve, where it aspirates blood from the left ventricle and propels it into the ascending aorta

Potential advantages of the Impella compared to the TandemHeart include miniature size (13 F versus 17 F), ease of insertion, maintenance of limb perfusion, and low bleeding rate. Retrograde insertion of the Impella is a technique familiar to most cardiologists. However, the Impella 2.5 can generate only 2.5 l of cardiac output and hence is suitable for patients with some intrinsic left ventricular function. The TandemHeart, however, can generate an output of 3.5 l/min and can almost completely replace left ventricle function.

The Impella is approved in Europe for left ventricle support for up to 5 days and has been used in a variety of conditions including acute heart failure, acute myocardial infarction, PCI, and during and after cardiac surgery (especially for postcardiotomy low cardiac output syndrome). In the United States, it is approved only for investigational use; a clinical trial (PROTECT 1) is underway to evaluate its use during high-risk percutaneous coronary intervention. Further studies will be done to determine the Impella's potential as a support device during cardiogenic shock.

Cancion Cardiac Recovery System

The Cancion® Cardiac Recovery System (Orqis Medical, Lake Forest, CA) (Fig. 6.3) is technically not a left ventricular support device. The Cancion pump is based on the principle of continuous aortic flow augmentation (CAFA), whereby, in animal models, providing additional continuous flow to the pulsatile aortic flow within the descending aorta resulted in ventricular unloading and improved hemodynamics [25]. Part of improved hemodynamics resulted from augmented renal perfusion. The inflow cannula is inserted in the femoral artery instead of the left atrium (as with the TandemHeart), obviating the need for transseptal puncture. The blood is returned to the descending aorta and blood flow within the aorta is augmented throughout the cardiac cycle. This device requires no mechanical connection to the heart. The pump itself is a frictionless magnetic levitation pump that is claimed to have a lower risk of thrombosis than the TandemHeart.

In an uncontrolled study of 24 patients with acute, decompensated heart failure unresponsive

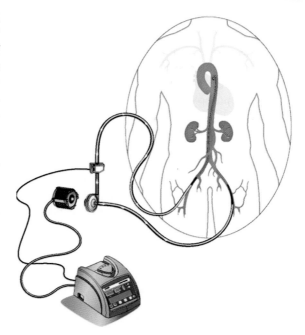

Fig. 6.3 Cancion cardiac recovery system

to medical therapy, the Cancion system decreased the pulmonary capillary wedge pressure, systemic vascular resistance, and serum creatinine level while improving the cardiac index [25]. This device is also currently undergoing clinical trials (MOMENTUM) to determine if short-term (4 days) support in refractory heart failure patients can lead to long-term benefits.

Percutaneous Long-Term Left Ventricular Support

Currently available devices are able to provide left ventricular support for a short duration only. Development of percutaneously or minimally invasive long-term support devices is also underway. At least three such devices are undergoing preclinical evaluation. The Synergy device (CircuLite, Inc., Hackensack, NJ) is being developed as a pocket circulatory assist (PAC) device that would sit in a subcuatenous pocket over the chest wall and use a micro-pump with cannulas in the subclavian artery and vein to withdraw blood from the left atrium through a transseptal approach and deliver it to the subclavian artery. The device is connected to a power supply via a percutaneous lead that exits the body in the abdominal area. Clinical evaluation of the Synergy device are anticipated to begin in the United States in 2008 [26]. The Exeleras System (Orqis Medical, Lake Forest, CA) is a longer duration version of the Cancion pump. It consists of a small implantable pump placed in an abdominal pocket and grafts that are connected to an iliac or femoral artery and tunneled to an axillary artery. A small percutaneous line leads to the external controller and battery pack. When activated, the system pumps blood from a patient's iliac artery into the descending aorta to provide CAFA. The Exeleras System is expected to enter clinical evaluation in 2008 [27].

Finally, at the Texas Heart Institute, we are developing a concept device that will consist of a catheter deployed micropump in the descending aorta and fixated with metallic struts to the aortic wall. It is designed to accelerate blood flow in the descending aorta to unload the heart. Its power will be supplied through a transarterial power cable to an outside power source. Though still in the conceptual phase only, it may be truly implantable in the cath lab without surgery.

Conclusions

Percutaneous left ventricular support therapy is an evolving field. Ongoing studies will establish the role of this therapy in the management of advanced congestive heart failure.

References

1. Jessup M, Brozena S. Heart failure. N Engl J Med 2003;348:2007–2018
2. Hosenpud JD, Bennett LE, Keck BM, Boucek MM, Novick RJ. The registry of the international society for heart and lung transplantation: seventeenth official report: 2000. J Heart Lung Transplan. 2000; 19: 909–931.
3. Kantrowitz A. Origins of intraaortic balloon pumping. Ann Thorac Surg 1990 Oct;50(4):672–674
4. Barron HV, Every NR, Parsons LS, et al. The use of intra-aortic balloon counterpulsation in patients with cardiogenic shock complicating acute myocardial infarction: data from the National Registry of Myocardial Infarction 2. Am Heart J 2001;141:933–939.
5. Scheidt S, Wilner G, Mueller H, Summers D, Lesch M, Wolff G, Krakauer J, Rubenfire M, Fleming P, Noon G, Oldham N, Killip T, Kantrowitz A. Intra-aortic balloon counterpulsation in cardiogenic shock: report of a cooperative clinical trial. N Engl Med 1973;288:979–984
6. Nanas JN, Moulopoulos SD. Counterpulsation: historical background, technical improvements, hemodynamic and metabolic effects. Cardiology 1994;84:156–167
7. Hochman JS, Sleeper LA, Webb JG, et al. Early revascularization in acute myocardial infarction complicated by cardiogenic shock. N Engl J Med 1999 Aug 26;341:625–634
8. Barron HV, Pirzada SR, Lomnitz DJ, Every NR, Gore JM, Chou TM. Use of intra-aortic balloon counterpulsation in patients with acute myocardial infarction complicated by cardiogenic shock. J Am Coll Cardiol 1998;31(Suppl A):135A–135A [abstract]
9. Thiele H, Lauer B, Hambrecht R, Boudriot E, Cohen HA, Schuler G. Reversal of cardiogenic shock by percutaneous left atrial-to-femoral arterial bypass assistance. Circulation 2001;104:2917–2922
10. Davies CH. Revascularization for cardiogenic shock. QJM 2001 Feb;94(2):57–67
11. Reynolds H, Hochman J. Cardiogenic shock: current concepts and improving outcomes. Circulation 2000 Feb 5;117(5):686–697
12. Wohlschlaeger J, Schmitz KJ, Schmid C, Schmid KW, Keul P, Takeda A, et al. Reverse remodeling following insertion of left ventricular assist devices (LVAD): a review of the morphological and molecular changes. Cardiovasc Res 2005;68:376–386.
13. Dipla K, Mattiello JA, Jeevanandum V, Houser SR, Margulies KB. Myocyte recovery after mechanical circulatory support in humans with end-stage heart failure. Circulation 1998;97:2316–2322
14. Zafeiridis A, Jeevanandam V, Houser SR, Margulies KB. Regression of cellular hypertrophy after left ventricular assist device support. Circulation 1998;98:656–662
15. Barbone A, Holmes JW, Heerdt PM, The' AH, Naka Y, Joshi N, Daines M, Marks AR, Oz MC, Burkhoff D. Comparison of right and left ventricular responses to left ventricular assist device support in patients with severe heart failure: a primary role of mechanical unloading underlying reverse remodeling. Circulation 2001;104:670–675
16. Hetzer R, Muller JH, Weng YG, Loebe M, Wallukat G. Midterm follow-up of patients who underwent removal of a left ventricular assist device after cardiac recovery from end-stage dilated cardiomyopathy. J Thorac Cardiovasc Surg 2000;120:843–853
17. Maybaum S, Mancini D, Xydas S, Starling RC, Aaronson K, Pagani FD, Miller LW, Margulies K, McRee S, Frazier OH, Torre-Amione G, LVAD Working Group. Cardiac improvement during mechanical circulatory support: a prospective multicenter study of the LVAD Working Group. Circulation 2007 May 15;115(19):2497–505. Epub 2007 May 7
18. Yacoub MH. A novel strategy to maximize the efficacy of left ventricular assist devices as a bridge to recovery. Eur Heart J 2001;22:534–540

19. Michael S. Lee MDa, Raj R, Makkar MD. Percutaneous left ventricular support devices. Cardiol Clin 2006 May; 24(2):265–275

20. Stephan W, Bernhard M. Impella assisted high risk percutaneous coronary intervention. Kardiovaskuläre Medizin 2005;8:187–189

21. Burkhoff D, Cohen H, Brunckhorst C, O'Neill WW. A randomized multicenter clinical study to evaluate the safety and efficacy of the TandemHeart percutaneous ventricular assist device versus conventional therapy with intraaortic balloon pumping for treatment of cardiogenic shock. Am Heart J 2006;152:469e1–469e8

22. Vranckx P, Foley DP, Feijter PJ, Vos J, Smits P, Serruys PW. Clinical introduction of the Tandemheart, a percutaneous left ventricular assist device, for circulatory support during high-risk percutaneous coronary intervention. Internat J Cardiovasc Intervent 2003;5:35–39

23. Meyns B, Stolinski J, Leunens V, et al., Left ventricular support by catheter-mounted axial flow pump reduces infarct size. J Am Coll Cardiol 2003;41:1087–1095)

24. Meyns B, Dens J, Sergeant P, et al., Initial experiences with the Impella-device in patients with cardiogenic shock. Thorac Cardio Surg 2003;51:1–6

25. Konstam MA, Czerska B, Bohm M, Oren RM, Sadowski J, Khanal S, Abraham T, Wasler A, Dahm JB, Gavazzi A, Gradinac S, Legrand V, Mohacsi P, Poelzl G, Radovancevic B, Van Bakel AB, Zile MR, Cabuay B, Bartus K, Jansen P. Aortic flow augmentation: a pilot study of hemodynamic and renal responses to a novel percutaneous intervention in decompensated heart failure. Circulation 2005;112:3107–3114.

26. Courtesy of Circulite website: http://www.circulite.net/about_us/faq

27. Courtesy of Orquis Systems website: http://www.orqis.com/exeleras.php

Chapter 7
Cellular Implantation Therapy

Current Studies, Different Strategies and Potential Applications

Emerson C. Perin, Guilherme V. Silva and James T. Willerson

Introduction

Acute myocardial infarction (AMI) may cause varying degrees of damage to the myocardium, depending on the amount of necrosis and the patency of the arterial bed. Myocardial scarring may compromise myocardial performance, leading to left ventricular remodeling in response to increased mechanical wall stress, inadequate perfusion that compromises remaining viable myocardial segments, and, finally, ischemic heart failure.

Despite efforts such as revascularization to halt the progression to ischemic heart failure, ventricular remodeling is still a growing danger. Efforts to treat severely failing hearts refractory to medical therapy have included heart transplantation and mechanical ventricular assistance [1]. Until recently, cardiologists believed that beyond revascularization and medical therapy, the process of ischemic heart failure was irreversible because the heart lacked the capacity to renew itself.

However, new insights into the mechanisms of cardiac repair have provided evidence that the adult heart can at least partially repair injury and that vasculogenesis may not occur solely during embryonic development. These insights, in turn, have sparked strong interest in the field of stem cell therapy [2, 3]. Prompted by evidence that adult bone marrow harbors a reservoir of plastic cells [4], animal experiments have generated evidence

supporting the use of stem cells for repairing cardiac tissue in diverse clinical settings [5].

The idea of using stem cells for cardiac repair by replacing or healing myocardium has been met both with enthusiasm and skepticism. There are several areas that are controversial and many basic mechanistic questions related to stem cell biology have yet to be answered. Although some of the body's natural healing responses are being elucidated, the main pathways of heart self-regeneration remain unclear. Meanwhile, clinical researchers, who face daily the challenge of a growing number of patients with severe coronary artery disease (CAD) and heart failure, have started to pursue venues in human clinical experimentation with stem cell therapy. In turn, stem cell therapy for cardiac diseases is becoming a clinical reality. Several strategies have been tested with promising initial results. This chapter is directed at the clinical cardiologist who will ultimately deliver this investigational therapy to patients. In this chapter, we outline basic concepts of stem cell therapy and review clinical data from phase I/II trials.

Stem Cell Basics

Definition

Stem cells are self-replicating cells capable of generating, sustaining, and replacing terminally differentiated cells [6, 7]. Stem cells can be subdivided into two large groups: embryonic and adult. Embryonic

E.C. Perin (✉)
Stem Cell Center, Texas Heart Institute, St. Luke's Episcopal Hospital, Houston, TX 77030, USA
e-mail: eperin@crescentb.net

R. Delgado, H.S. Arora (eds.), *Interventional Treatment of Advanced Ischemic Heart Disease*,
DOI 10.1007/978-1-84800-395-8_7, © Springer-Verlag London Limited 2009

stem cells are present in the earliest stage of embryonic development$^3/_4$the blastocyst. Embryonic stem cells are pluripotent, meaning they are capable of generating any terminally differentiated cell in the human body that is derived from any one of the three embryonic germ layers: ectoderm, mesoderm, or endoderm [8]. All the body's organs arise through a series of divisions and differentiations from the original embryonic stem cells that form the blastocyst [3].

Adult stem cells are intrinsic to specific tissues of the postnatal organism and are committed to differentiate into those tissues [9]. Adult stem cells yield mature differentiated cells capable of performing the specialized function(s) of that tissue in helping to maintain organ homeostasis. Each type of differentiated cell has its own phenotype, including shape or morphology; interactions with surrounding cells and extracellular matrix; expression of cell surface proteins (receptors); and biological behavior [8]. Adult tissue-specific stem cells are present in self-renewable organs, including the liver, pancreas, skeletal muscle, skin, and heart.

Stem Cell Identification

Each adult stem cell subtype can be identified by cell surface receptors that selectively bind to particular signaling molecules. Differences in structure and binding affinity allow for a remarkable multiplicity of receptors. Normally, cells utilize these receptors and the molecules that bind to them to communicate with other cells and perform the proper function of the tissue to which they belong (e.g., contraction, secretion, synaptic transmission). Each type of adult stem cell has a certain receptor or combination of receptors (i.e., marker) that distinguishes it from other types of stem cells (Table 7.1).

Stem cell markers are often given letter and number codes based on the molecules that bind to them (Table 7.1). A cell presenting the stem cell antigen-1 receptor is identified as Sca-1$^+$. Cells exhibiting Sca-1 but not CD34 antigen or lineage-specific antigen (Lin) are identified as CD34$^-$Sca-1$^+$Lin$^-$. This particular combination of surface receptors identifies mesenchymal stem cells (MSCs).

Table 7.1 Conditions, drugs, and cytokines that may affect number and function of human EPCs

Condition or factor	Changes in number/function of EPCs or CD34$^+$cells	Investigators
Physiological		
Gender (e.g., estrogens)	↑ CD34$^+$/VEGFR2$^+$ cells	Strehlow et al. [156]
Physical training	↑ EPC number	Adams et al. [157]
Pathological		
Coronary artery disease/number of risk factors	↓ EPC number and migration	Vasa et al. [31]
Smoking	↓ CD34$^+$/KDR$^+$ cells	
	↓ EPCs or CD34$^+$/KDR$^+$ cells	
Family history	↓ EPCs or CD34$^+$/KDR$^+$ cells	
Hypertension	↓ EPC migration	
Cumulative cardiovascular risk factor score	↓ EPC CFUs	Hill et al. [119]
Myocardial infarction	↑ CD34$^+$ cells	Shintani et al. [3]
	↑ CD34$^+$/ACC133$^+$/VEGFR2$^+$ cells	
Vascular injury	↑ ACC133$^+$/ VEGFR2$^+$ cells	Gill et al. [16]
Congestive heart failure (class I–II)	↑ CD34$^+$ cells	Valgimigli et al. [158]
	↑ CD34$^+$/ACC133$^+$/VEGFR2$^+$ cells	
	↑ EPC CFUs	
Congestive heart failure (class III–IV)	↓ CD34$^+$ cells	
	↓ CD34$^+$/ACC133$^+$/VEGFR2$^+$ cells	
	↓ EPC CFUs	
In-stent restenosis	↓ EPC CFUs	George et al. [159]
	↓ EPC adhesion	
Drugs and cytokines		
HMG-CoA reductase inhibitors	↑ EPC number	Dimmeler et al. [160]
G-CSF	↑ CD133$^+$/VEGFR2$^+$ cells	Peichev et al. [25]
Erythropoietin	↑ CD34$^+$/CD45$^+$ cells	Bahlmann et al. [161]

Reprinted from [167] with permission.

Unfortunately, the identification of stem cells solely on the basis of cell surface markers has led to confusion. Surface markers have long been used in the hematology literature but provide for inexact and precise identification of stem cell subpopulations given the plasticity of stem cells. In addition the cell surface markers' nomenclature can be confusing. Various investigators have given the same bone marrow cells different names. In some cases, surface marker designations within cell subtypes overlap. Most surface markers do not adequately identify stem cells because they may also be found on non-stem cells. Moreover, some markers may be expressed only under certain culture conditions or at certain stages of cell development.

Newer strategies for stem cell identification have been developed based on the knowledge of cell functions. A primitive and multipotential subpopulation of bone marrow mononuclear cells has been identified on the basis of the intracellular presence of aldehyde dehydrogenase (ALDH). Those cells can be "marked" on the basis of the presence of ALDH and are called aldehyde dehydrogenase-bright cells (ALDH[br] cells), allowing for their separation from a bone marrow aspiration mononuclear subpopulation under fluorescence-activated cell sorter (FACS) analysis.

Thus, cell surface markers remain a useful tool and have widespread use, as evidenced by the stem cell literature. Limitations, explained in the bone marrow transplantation literature, highlight the need for the development of new methods for identifying stem cells in the emerging field of cell therapy for cardiac diseases. Indeed, functional assays will likely play an important role in stem cell selection and classification in the future.

Postnatal Vasculogenesis: Stem Cells and Vascular Repair

The field of stem cell therapy has benefited from the work of numerous basic and clinical scientists whose studies have greatly improved our understanding of the processes involved in cardiac repair and neovascularization. The creation of new blood vessels (neovascularization) requires the formation of new mature endothelial cells. In this process, the new endothelial cells migrate or proliferate from existing vessels (angiogenesis) or arise from bone marrow-derived progenitor cells to generate new vessels (vasculogenesis) [10]. Asahara et al. [2] were the first to describe a unique population of bone marrow-derived endothelial progenitor cells (EPCs) found in the peripheral circulation. These EPCs have certain functional similarities with bone marrow hematopoietic progenitor cells (HPCs). Before EPCs were discovered, vasculogenesis was thought to occur only in the human embryonic phase. However, in animal models of ischemia, EPCs participate in the development of new vessels, thus establishing a new paradigm of postnatal vasculogenesis [11–30].

The importance of postnatal vasculogenesis to stem cell therapy has been highlighted in several recent studies. Bone marrow-derived EPCs have been shown to contribute functionally to vasculogenesis after AMI [1, 13, 14], in wound healing [31], and in limb ischemia [12–14, 19, 20, 27, 30]. They have also been implicated in the endothelialization of vascular grafts [13, 21, 28]. The number of circulating EPCs and their migratory capacity correlates inversely with risk factors for CAD, such as smoking and hypercholesterolemia [31]. EPCs have also been implicated in the pathogenesis of allograft transplant vasculopathy and coronary restenosis after stent placement, after being recruited by appropriate cytokines, growth factors, and hormones via autocrine, paracrine, and endocrine mechanisms [32]. Endothelial progenitor cell mobilization is a natural response to vascular trauma, as seen in patients who undergo coronary artery bypass surgery or suffer burns [16] or an AMI [1].

Stem Cells and Cardiac Repair

Adult tissue-specific stem cells are present in other self-renewable organs, including the liver, pancreas, skeletal muscle, and skin. The heart, which until very recently was considered a terminally differentiated, postmitotic organ with a finite store of myocytes established at birth, may now be added to this list. It has recently been observed that hematopoietic stem cells (HSCs) can transdifferentiate into cardiomyocytes [33, 34] and that stem cells reside in the heart [35]. These resident cardiac stem cells (CSCs) appear to occupy niches in the atria and apex and have been observed in the border zones of myocardial infarcts [36, 37]. Such observations have, in turn, drastically changed our understanding of the cardiac repair process. Now it appears that resident CSCs and possibly bone marrow-derived stem cells may be able to help repair damaged hearts. Once adequate signaling is established with cytokines and growth factors, bone marrow cells are mobilized [32]. Strengthening this concept is evidence from animal studies showing that AMI repair involves bone marrow cells [38] and by evidence of chimerism in transplanted hearts [39].

Further evidence for a dynamic cardiac renewal process in the adult heart comes from the recent identification of a novel population of early tissue-committed stem cells that may be part of a group of circulating progenitor cells involved in cardiac repair [40].

Atherosclerosis and the Senescent Bone Marrow Hypothesis

Evidence also suggests that stem cells play key roles in the adult heart's ability to dynamically repair itself and its vessels and in the body's ability to maintain vascular homeostasis.

Studies by several research groups have shown that cells derived from bone marrow accelerate the re-endothelization process [41]. Evidence has also emerged suggesting that the presence of risk factors and the aging process can lead to bone marrow failure and the depletion of progenitor cells needed for vascular repair. This may also be true in inflammatory states, such as diabetes mellitus and CAD. Fadini et al. [42] have demonstrated decreased EPC levels in patients with diabetes. They hypothesize that the depletion of circulating EPCs in diabetic patients may be involved in the pathogenesis of peripheral vascular complications [42]. Walter et al. [43] have demonstrated that the reduced neovascularization capacity of EPCs in patients with CAD derives from an impaired CXCR4 signaling pathway. CXCR4 is a cytokine receptor essential for the migration and homing of HSCs.

Dong et al. [44] have summarized the role of bone marrow in vascular repair. In the presence of competent bone marrow, the inflammatory signals (cytokines, etc.) generated by vascular injury result in the recruitment of bone marrow progenitor cells capable of assisting in arterial repair, thus providing a negative feedback loop that, in turn, shuts down the production of inflammatory mediators leading to homeostasis (Fig. 7.1). By contrast, in the presence of a senescent bone marrow, the inflammatory signals do not result in mobilization of progenitor cells capable of healing. Instead, progressive atherosclerosis and further injury by amplification of the inflammatory signaling may occur. Inflammation in itself has been shown to create vascular injury that perpetuates the disease state.

Stem Cells as Biomarkers

As mentioned above, EPCs appear to be important in vascular homeostasis [44]. Accordingly, Werner

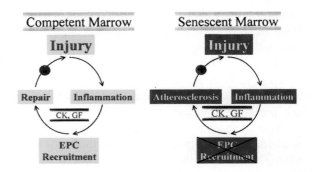

Fig. 7.1 Effect of bone marrow obsolescence on arterial repair and inflammation. In the presence of a competent bone marrow capable of producing the type of progenitor cells for arterial repair (young marrow), inflammatory cytokines, growth factors, and other agonists contribute to the recruitment of repair cells. Once the arterial lesion is repaired successfully, the inflammatory markers subside (negative feedback loop). In contrast, if the bone marrow is unable to produce these progenitor cells, either because the pathways that are required for their production are deficient or because the produced cells are somehow incompetent, the inflammatory factors continue to increase, essentially indicating a persistent arterial lesion. The increase in inflammatory factors, in turn, can further promote arterial damage, with worsening of atherosclerosis and destabilization of atherosclerotic plaques (positive feedback loop). CK, cytokines and other inflammation agonists; EPC, endothelial progenitor cell; GF, growth factors. (Adapted from Goldschmidt-Clermont et al. [166]) Reprinted from [44]

et al.'s [45] series of 519 CAD patients followed-up for up to 1 year after coronary angiography found that preprocedural EPC levels are prognostically valuable in predicting death from cardiovascular causes and major cardiovascular events (MACE). Patients with higher EPC levels appear to be less likely to suffer these untoward events, even after adjustment for traditional prognostic and risk factors.

Schmidt-Lucke et al. [46] followed 120 patients (43 control subjects, 44 patients with stable CAD, and 33 patients with acute coronary syndromes) for 10 months and recorded MACE events (Fig. 7.2). Patients with reduced EPCs had significantly higher rates of MACE. When the results were analyzed by multivariate analysis, reduced EPC levels were found to be an independent predictor of worse prognosis, even after adjustment for traditional cardiovascular risk factors and disease activity (hazard ratio, 3.9; $P < 0.05$).

This preliminary evidence suggests a possible role of circulating stem cell subpopulations as biomarkers. EPCs might provide a unique window into patients' vascular health. Moreover, functional studies, such as stromal-derived factor 1 (SDF-1) migratory capacity, may add a more powerful predictive value to the absolute number of EPCs.

Currently, the utilization of EPCs as biomarkers is premature, and their clinical usefulness in that capacity will require examination in larger studies in multiple clinical scenarios and in broader patient populations.

Stem Cell Types and Characteristics

Adult Bone Marrow-Derived Stem Cells

Adult bone marrow-derived stem cells are presently the cell types most widely utilized in cardiac stem cell therapy. A heterogeneous subset, termed autologous bone marrow-derived mononuclear cells (ABMMNCs), is composed of small amounts of stromal or MSCs, HPCs, EPCs, and more committed cell lineages, such as natural killer lymphocytes, T lymphocytes, B lymphocytes, and others [2].

Bone marrow stem cells are aspirated from the patient's iliac crest under local anesthesia. The

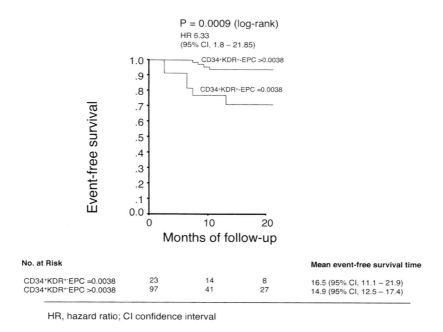

HR, hazard ratio; CI confidence interval

Fig. 7.2 Event-free survival according to levels of circulating CD34$^+$KDR$^+$-EPCs defined by ROC curve analysis. Reprinted from [46]

mononuclear subfraction of the aspirate is isolated by means of Ficoll density centrifugation, filtered through a 100-μm nylon mesh to remove cell aggregates or bone spicules, and washed several times in phospate-buffered saline solution before being used immediately for therapy or expanded in an endothelial cell-specific culture medium. EPCs can be harvested from peripheral blood.

Thus far, the most important bone marrow subtypes utilized for cardiac repair have been MSCs, EPCs, or, alternatively, the whole ABMMNC fraction. Newly described bone marrow cell subtypes with therapeutic potential are discussed below.

Mesenchymal Stem Cells

Adult MSCs are cells from any adult tissue that can be expanded in culture and renew themselves and differentiate into several specific mesenchymal cell lineages. MSCs are present in different niches throughout the body, such as bone marrow and adipose tissue [47]. MSCs are extremely plastic, with the potential to terminally differentiate in vitro and in vivo into mesenchymal phenotypes, such as bone [48, 49], cartilage [50], tendon [51, 52], muscle [33, 53], adipose tissue [54, 55], and hematopoiesis-supporting stroma [50]. MSCs differentiate not only into mesenchymal tissues but also into cells derived from other embryonic layers, including neurons [56] and epithelia in the skin, lung, liver, intestine, kidney, and spleen [57–59]. Their plasticity has increased interest in using them for cardiac regeneration.

In a proof-of-concept study in which Saito et al. [60] intravenously injected LacZ reporter gene-transfected MSCs into healthy rats, the MSCs preferentially engrafted in the bone marrow. When injected into rats subjected to repetitive periods of ischemia/reperfusion, however, the MSCs engrafted in the infarcted regions of the heart, where they participated in angiogenesis and expressed cardiomyocyte-specific proteins. When injected into rats 10 days after myocardial injury, MSCs preferentially homed to damaged myocardium.

Mesenchymal stem cells are $CD45^-CD34^-$ bone marrow cells that can be readily grown in culture. They are rare in the bone marrow (<0.01% of nucleated cells, by some estimates) and thus ten times less abundant than HSCs. MSCs need to be cultured for at least 20 days to obtain necessary numbers for therapy, which directly affects clinical strategies for treating AMI that involves autologous MSCs.

Adult bone marrow MSCs, which are easy to manipulate genetically and weakly immunogenic, represent another potential source of allogeneic stem cells [61]. Allogeneic MSCs actually inhibit T cells in culture [62], and several in vivo studies have achieved good engraftment of allogeneic MSCs without rejection [61].

Our group at the Texas Heart Institute was the first to study mesenchymal cell injections in a large-animal model of chronic myocardial ischemia [63]. In brief, we used ameroid constrictors to induce ischemia in 12 mongrel dogs. One month later, we directly injected the myocardium of each dog with 100 million MSCs or saline as a control. Subsequent two-dimensional echocardiography showed improved systolic function both at rest and during stress in the treated animals (Fig. 7.3). Histopathologic studies showed that the MSCs had transdifferentiated into smooth muscle and endothelial cells (Figs. 7.4 and 7.5) and improved vascularization (Fig. 7.6).

Genetically modified MSCs have been preliminarily tested as an alternative therapeutic strategy. Genetically modified MSCs should, in theory, overcome one of the drawbacks of cell therapy: short-term survival of stem cells. Furthermore, these cells could potentially be used as "couriers" to deliver genes or as a factory by encoding genes that would secrete key substances to enhance angiogenesis (e.g., vascular endothelial growth factor [VEGF]).

Mangi et al. [64] have provided evidence of the in vivo efficacy of genetically modified MSCs. MSCs over-expressing the anti-apoptotic gene AKT-1 are more resistant to apoptosis in vitro and in vivo, limit ventricular remodeling, and improve cardiac function when injected into infarcted experimental animal hearts. Further adding to the prospects of genetically modified MSCs is work from Tang et al. [65]. In their experiments, MSCs transduced with heme-oxygenase (HO)-1 had better survival than did nonmodified MSCs and provided better healing after AMI in experimental animal models. Further work is needed to confirm the potential for genetically modified cells and their safety in larger

A

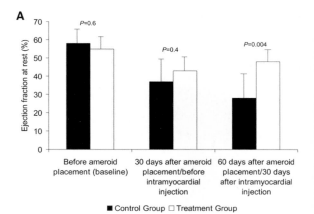

B

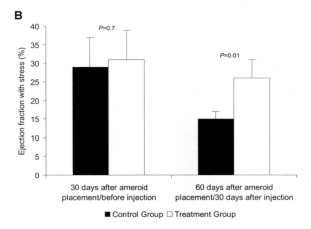

Fig. 7.3 (A) Left ventricular ejection fraction at rest. Assessments were made at baseline before ameroid placement (*left*), 30 days later at time of cell or saline injection (*middle*), and 60 days after ameroid placement (*right*). (B) Left ventricular ejection fraction with stress. Assessments were made before and 30 days after intramyocardial injection. Reprinted from [63]

animal models before phase I clinical trials can begin. In light of the current evidence, however, MSCs should have strong clinical potential, especially if human safety studies confirm the lack of rejection demonstrated thus far in preclinical studies.

Endothelial Progenitor Cells

Endothelial progenitor cells can be isolated from the mononuclear fraction of the bone marrow or peripheral blood, as well as from fetal liver or umbilical cord blood [12, 23, 66, 67]. Heterologous,

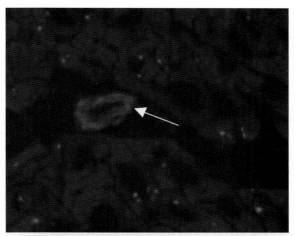

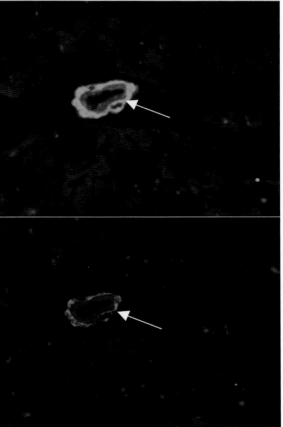

Fig. 7.4 (*Top*) DiI-positive stem cells (red) in the midmyocardium of the anterolateral wall. (*Middle*) α-Smooth muscle actin staining with FITC (*green*) showing cross-section of vessel wall. (*Bottom*) Stained areas show colocalization (*yellow*) of stem cells and smooth muscle cells, suggesting transformation of stem cells into smooth muscle cells. The vessel shown is in the myocardial interstitium. Arrows point to vessel media. Reprinted from [63]

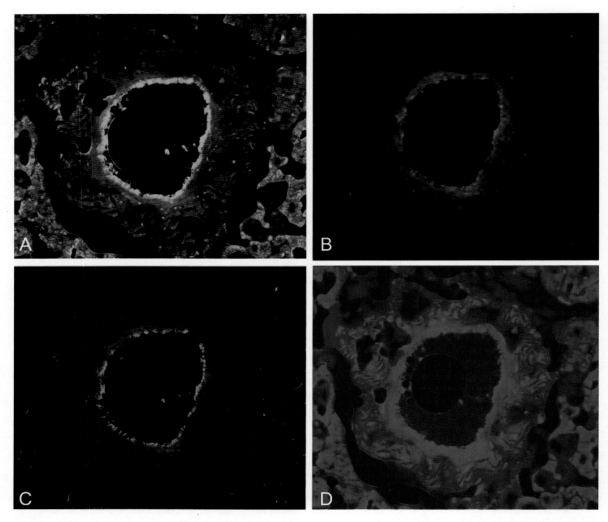

Fig. 7.5 (**A**) Factor VIII staining with FITC (green) showing a thin vessel wall. (**B**) DiI-positive mesenchymal stem cells (red) in a vessel of the anterolateral wall. (**C**) Colocalization (yellow) of MSCs and endothelial cells, indicating transformation of MSCs into endothelial cells. (**D**) DAPI stain showing labeled endothelial nuclei. Reprinted from [63]

homologous, and autologous EPCs have been shown to engraft at sites of active neovascularization in widely ranging animal models of ischemia [67].

EPCs can differentiate into endothelial cells, smooth muscle cells, or cardiomyocytes, both in vitro and in vivo. EPCs have been identified by different research groups using different methodologies [15, 17, 22, 25]. The classic methods involve culture of total peripheral blood mononuclear cells or isolation via magnetic microbeads coated with anti-CD133 or anti-CD34 antibodies. After isolation, the cells are cultured in a medium containing specific growth factors, such as VEGF and fibroblast growth factor, to facilitate the growth of endothelial-like cells.

"Immature" or "primitive" EPCs have a profile similar to that of HSCs: both cell types are thought to result from a common precursor, the hemangioblast. Within the bone marrow, immature EPCs and HSCs share common cell-surface markers: CD34, CD133, and VEGF receptor 2 (VEGFR-2, also known as KDR/FLK-1). Similarly, in the peripheral circulation, the more primitive cell population with the capacity of differentiating into EPCs expresses CD34, VEGFR-2, and CD133. In the peripheral circulation, the more committed EPCs

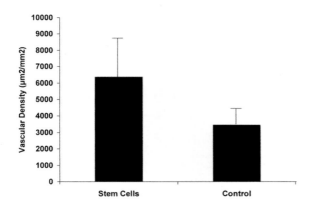

Fig. 7.6 Vascular density was statistically greater in the anterolateral walls of animals that received the stem cells. Reprinted from [63]

lose CD133 but retain CD34 and VEGFR-2 expression. Some circulating EPCs and, to a greater extent, more differentiated EPCs start expressing the endothelial lineage-specific marker vascular endothelial (VE) cadherin or E-selectin. However, when immature EPCs follow the hematopoietic path, the surface markers of CD133 and VEGFR-2 are extinguished because stem/progenitor cell markers are not expressed on differentiated hematopoietic cells (Fig. 7.7).

Recent studies have challenged traditional views that primitive bone marrow-derived EPCs that lose their CD133 marker become relatively committed EPCs that may subsequently differentiate into mature endothelial cells. EPCs (CD34/VEGF-2$^+$ cells) appear to originate from peripheral blood mononuclear cells that express the monocyte/macrophage markers CD14, MAC-1, and CD11-c, suggesting a possible monocyte/macrophage origin [68]. Harraz et al. [69] have observed, within populations of mononuclear peripheral cells, CD34$^-$ cells that are not only CD14$^+$ but also differentiate into endothelial cells. Adding to the debate is the recent description of "late" EPCs or outgrowth endothelial cells (OECs) that originate from a CD14$^-$ monocyte population [70]. EPCs originating from the CD14$^+$ monocyte population (so-called "early" EPCs) were found to secrete angiogenic peptides, such as VEGF, IL-8, and enzymes, including metalloproteinase (MMP) 9. However, these "early" EPCs did not proliferate well. On the other hand, OECs did proliferate well but secreted only MMP2. Taken together, these findings argue for the plasticity of EPCs (CD34$^+$, VEGFR-2$^+$, and CD133$^+$), the different developmental stages of a common precursor progenitor cell, and the existence of distinct cell subtypes that might be further differentiated by surface markers yet to be discovered.

Endothelial progenitor cell numbers appear to decrease in the presence of risk factors for CAD and to correlate negatively with Framingham cardiovascular risk factors [31]. Therefore, stem cell therapy with EPCs may prove very useful in the clinical setting of cardiovascular disease. The kinetic and biological properties of EPCs may be especially appropriate for autologous transplantation. EPCs may also be safe to use in elderly and diabetic patients, populations in which they do not tend to migrate as much or induce neovascularization [68].

Our ability to characterize EPCs and identify those subtypes most useful for cardiac cell therapy has advanced rapidly but is still incomplete. Nonetheless, as the positive results of initial preclinical and clinical studies have shown, EPCs show great therapeutic promise.

Other Bone Marrow Stem Cells

Clearly, the bone marrow is a reservoir of cells whose regenerative capacity extends beyond the hematopoietic lineage. Identifying stem cells on the basis of cell-surface markers is a limited method that may delay the discovery of additional tissue-specific stem cell subtypes. Nevertheless, the stem cell field is advancing quickly. Recently, Kucia et al. [71] published the first evidence that postnatal bone marrow harbors a nonhematopoietic cell population that expresses markers for cardiac differentiation. This finding corroborates the early work of Deb et al. [72], who isolated Y-chromosome-positive cardiac myocytes from female recipients of male bone marrow. The percentage of cardiomyocytes that harbored the Y chromosome was quite small (only 0.23%), but there was no evidence of either pseudonuclei or cell fusion. Two new bone marrow cardiac precursors have been identified: ABMMNCs expressing cardiac markers within a population of nonhematopoietic CXCR4$^+$/Sca-1$^+$/Lin$^-$/CD45$^-$ ABMMNCs in mice and within a population of

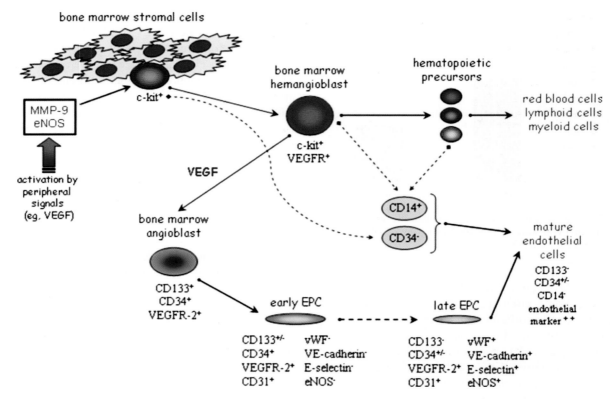

Fig. 7.7 Mobilization, recruitment, and differentiation of human bone marrow-derived angiogenic progenitor cells. Initial step in the recruitment of angiogenic stem/progenitor cells from the bone marrow represents the activation of matrix metalloproteinase-9 (MMP-9), which promotes the transformation of membrane bound Kit-ligand to a soluble Kit-ligand. This activation is followed by detachment of early cKit[+] progenitor cells from the bone marrow stromal niche and their subsequent movement to the vascular zone of the bone marrow. An important regulator of this mobilization is VEGF, which binds to its receptor VEGFR-2, thus mediating the further maturation of the cascade hemangioblast–angioblast–early EPC–late EPC.

Bone marrow-derived endothelial progenitor cells (EPCs) are of hematopoietic origin and possibly derive from the hemangioblast. These early progenitors (CD133[+]/CD34[+]/VEGFR-2[+]/CD14[-]) represent a small population with proliferative potential, capable to give rise to late endothelial outgrowth. Cells of myeloid origin (CD14[+]) may also trans- ifferentiate into endothelial cells and secret angiogenic factors, but their proliferative potential is limited and they did not generate a stable late outgrowth. Mesenchymal CD34[-] progenitor cells can also generate endothelial cells; however, these cells showed in vivo reduced functional activity and incorporation into neo-vessels. Reprinted from [167]

nonhematopoietic CXCR4[+]/CD34[+]/AC133[+]/CD45[-] ABMMNCs in humans. These nonhematopoietic ABMMNCs expressing cardiac precursors are mobilized into the peripheral blood after a myocardial infarction and home to the damaged myocardium in an SDF-1-CXCR4-, HGF-c-Met-, and LIF-LIF-R-dependent manner [71].

The identification of a direct cardiac precursor within the bone marrow cell population opens up a vast number of possibilities for the field of cardiac regeneration. In theory, in vitro expansion of this type of cell would be therapeutically attractive.

Skeletal Myoblasts

Skeletal myoblasts are adult, tissue-specific stem cells [73] located between the basal lamina and the sarcolemma on the periphery of the mature skeletal-muscle fiber [74]. Also known as muscle satellite cells, these small, mononuclear cells are activated by biochemical signals to divide and differentiate into fusion-competent cells after muscle injury.

The use of skeletal myoblasts for cardiac repair originated from earlier attempts where fetal cardiomyocytes were used. When injected into the border zone of an AMI, fetal cardiomyocytes can engraft and survive [75]. Despite initial encouraging results in animal models, however, clinical use of fetal cardiomyocytes has not been pursued in the United States presently because of ethical issues and the limited availability of these cells.

Skeletal myoblasts are viewed as an attractive alternative by some [76]. The first therapeutic trials used skeletal myoblasts obtained under sterile conditions and local anesthesia from 0.5- to 5.0-g muscle biopsy specimens. Individual cells were isolated by digestion with trypsin and collagenase, washed to remove red blood cells and debris, plated, and cultured to obtain the numbers necessary for therapeutic use.

Skeletal myoblasts can survive prolonged periods of hypoxia [77]. Like fetal cardiomyocytes, skeletal myoblasts survive and may engraft (although this is controversial) when injected into the border zone of an AMI.

Embryonic Stem Cells

As gradually revealed over the past two decades, ESCs are derived from the cell mass of blastocysts in mice and humans. In the presence of leukemia inhibitory factor (LIF) or in a layer of mitotically inactivated mouse embryonic fibroblasts, ESCs proliferate indefinitely. Once removed from these conditions and transferred into a suspension culture, ESCs spontaneously form multicellular aggregates that turn into endoderm, mesoderm, and ectoderm [77]. Murine ESC lines have been shown in vitro to differentiate into cells (hematopoietic progenitors, adipocytes, hepatocytes, smooth muscle cells, endothelial cells, neurons, and others) associated with each of the three layers [78, 79]. More importantly, they have been shown to differentiate into cardiomyocytes [80] in response to appropriate stimuli and specific signaling factors. Hepatocyte growth factor (HGF), epidermal growth factor (EGF), basic fibroblast growth factor (bFGF), platelet-derived growth factor (PDGF), retinoic acid, vitamin C, and overexpression of GAT4 all enhance this differentiation process in vitro [81]. However, the ideal combination of these factors for enhancing ESC differentiation into cardiomyocytes remains unknown.

Because ESCs are pluripotent and can proliferate indefinitely, they may have an important potential role in cardiac regeneration. Although ethical issues involving the use of human ESCs has slowed research in several countries, including the United States, enthusiasm about their future clinical utilization remains high.

Resident Cardiac Stem Cells

Myocyte replication is the failing heart's attempt to compensate for a limited capacity for hypertrophy. When Urbanek et al. [37] used Ki-67 (a nuclear protein expressed during cell division) to assess the mitotic activity of myocytes, they observed significantly greater mitotic activity at infarct border zones than in distant myocardium or undiseased control hearts. The evidence that cardiac myocytes divide shortly after a myocardial infarction led investigators to search for the origin of the dividing myocytes [82]. This culminated in the description of resident CSCs [35–37].

The change in paradigm has provided a new insight into the heart's biology and mechanisms of repair: the heart has primitive cells that can generate new myocytes, smooth muscle cells, and endothelial cells (Fig. 7.8). New myocytes are generated throughout life, but it remains unclear why certain types of injury, such as after an AMI, are associated with incomplete healing. It has been shown, however, that CSCs can be coaxed to repair injured areas [83].

Resident CSCs were first isolated in murine hearts. Characterization of these cells was based on the expression of the stem cell-related surface antigens c-Kit and Sca-1. In the first study, freshly isolated c-Kit$^+$/Lin$^-$ cells were shown to be clonogenic and to differentiate into myocytes, smooth muscle cells, and endothelial lineage cells [35]. Those cells generated functional myocardium when injected into ischemic areas of the heart. The second study characterized CSCs as Sca-1/c-Kit$^-$. When treated in culture with 5-azacytidine, those cells differentiated into a myogenic lineage. Subsequently, intravenous injection of the cells in an ischemia/reperfusion model resulted in infarct healing with cardiomyocyte transdifferentiation

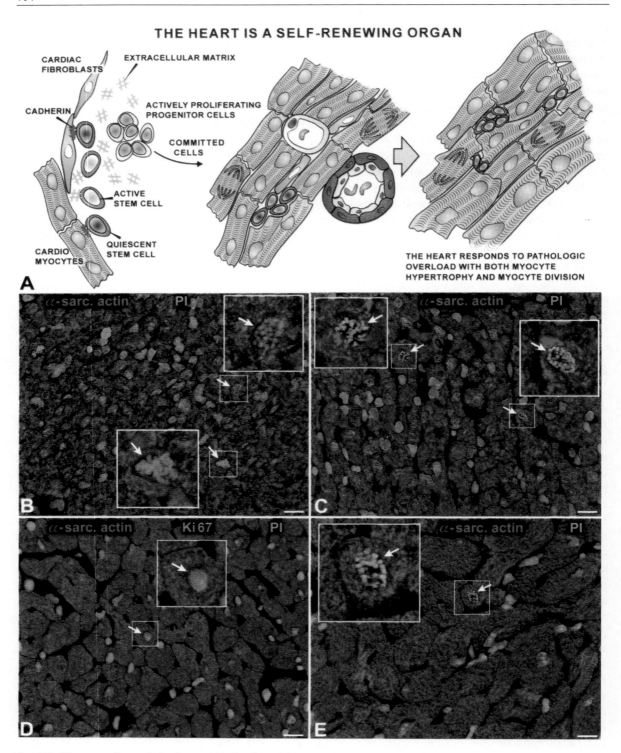

Fig. 7.8 New paradigm of the heart. (**A**) Cardiac niches contain stem cells, which, after activation, give rise to myocytes and vascular structures. (**B–E**) Dividing myocytes (α-sarcomeric actin, *red*) in fetal (**B**), neonatal (**C**), adult (**D**), and hypertrophied (**E**) rat heart. Mitotic myocytes (arrows) are shown in inserts. Bright blue denotes Ki67. Scale bars = 10 μm. Reprinted from [168]

[82]. In studies involving atrial and ventricular biopsies in sheep and humans, Messina et al. [84] isolated a cardiac progenitor cell that was c-Kit$^+$ and capable of self-proliferating into a large number of cells. The authors also showed that human CSCs could participate in infarct repair in the murine model.

The developing and adult heart has a cell pool that has been described as the CSC side-population pool. These cells share the ability to efflux Hoechst 33342 dye as the bone marrow side-population. Those cells are CD31$^+$, raising suspicion that they are of bone marrow origin rather than of true cardiac origin. Recently a SCA-1, CD31$^-$ cardiac SP has been identified; it has a high regenerative potential and is able to terminally differentiate into myocytes. Anversa et al. [82] have proposed a hierarchy of CSC growth and differentiation.

The current understanding of the biology of CSCs points to a homeostatic equilibrium of cell apoptosis and cell formation in normal hearts on the basis of the CSC compartment. Once disease ensues, such as chronic myopathic disease, this equilibrium is disrupted favoring apoptosis. It is unclear why the CSC pool also has limited regeneration capacity in the setting of acute myocardial injury. Future understanding of the biology of CSCs might provide better regenerative strategies after AMI and in the setting of chronic heart failure.

Alternative Sources of Stem Cells

Despite successful preclinical and clinical utilization of bone marrow cells and skeletal myoblasts, the search continues for an ethical, easily accessible, high-yield source of stem cells. MSCs have been isolated from adipose tissue, placental tissue, and umbilical cord blood. A number of studies have shown adipose-derived mesenchymal stem cells (AMSCs) to be pluripotent and capable of differentiating into multiple cell lineages along the myogenic, osteogenic, neurogenic, and hematopoietic pathways [85–87]. Additionally, AMSCs secrete VEGF, HGF, bFGF, and transforming growth factor beta (TGF-β), which have a potential angiogenic effect on ischemic myocardium [88]. These

cells also express the cell-surface marker CD34, but it is uncertain whether their pluripotency is limited to the subgroup of cells that express this marker [89]. Research to better characterize AMSCs and evaluate their safety and efficacy in preclinical studies is ongoing.

By means of dissection and proteinase digestion, large numbers of viable mononuclear cells can be harvested from the human placenta at term, and a mesenchymal cell population with characteristic expression of CD9, CD29, and CD73 can be obtained in culture. The in vitro growth behavior of such placenta-derived mesenchymal cells is similar to that of human bone marrow mesenchymal progenitor cells [90]. Transdifferentiation experiments have shown potential for differentiation along osteogenic, chondrogenic, adipogenic, and myogenic lines [90]. The human placenta at term might be an easily accessible, ample source of multipotent mesenchymal progenitor cells and is also under preclinical investigation.

Cord blood has long been used as a source of MSCs for bone marrow transplantation. The stem cell compartment is more abundant and less mature in cord blood than in bone marrow. Moreover, MSCs in cord blood have a higher proliferative potential because of their extended lifespan and longer telomeres [91–94]. Not only can cord-blood MSCs be harvested without morbidity to the donor, but they also display a robust in vitro capacity for directable or spontaneous differentiation into mesodermal, endodermal, and ectodermal cell fates. Cord-blood MSCs are CD45$^-$ and HLA-II$^-$ and can be expanded without losing their pluripotency. Therefore, cord blood is also undergoing preclinical evaluation as a possible easily accessible source of multipotent cells.

Stem Cell Delivery Methods

The current understanding of stem cell biology and kinetics gives important clues as to how one should deliver them. The efficacy of therapeutic stem cells will obviously depend largely on successful delivery. Stem cells have been delivered indirectly through peripheral and coronary veins and coronary arteries. Alternatively, they have been delivered directly by intramyocardial injections via surgical, transendocardial, or transvenous approaches. Another potential delivery strategy is the mobilization of stem cells from the bone marrow by means of cytokine therapy with or without peripheral harvesting.

The main objective of any cell delivery method is to achieve the concentration of stem cells necessary for repairing the damaged region being targeted. Toward this end, the ideal modality should be safe; easy to use; cost-effective; clinically useful in a wide range of clinical disease settings; easily, adequately, and effectively targeted; and able to exert a long-lasting therapeutic effect.

Stem Cell Mobilization

In humans, progenitor cells from the bone marrow mobilize after an AMI. This suggests a "natural" attempt at cardiac repair [3]. In theory, therapeutic mobilization of bone marrow progenitor cells after an AMI would amplify the existing healing response. Because of its simplicity, mobilization of stem cells is therefore an attractive delivery strategy [95–96]. It would not only obviate the need for invasive harvesting or delivery procedures, but also take advantage of the clinical procedures already established for the use of progenitor cell-mobilizing granulocyte colony-stimulating factor (G-CSF) in treating hematological disorders. However, because of the possibility of adverse events in a different patient population and the theoretical possibility of tumorigenesis, the safety of such "off-label" applications of G-CSF have been questioned.

Transvascular Delivery: Peripheral (Intravenous) Infusion

Peripheral (intravenous) infusion of stem cells as performed in bone marrow transplantation would be a very convenient—not to mention simple, widely available, and inexpensive—way of delivering therapeutic stem cells to myocardial targets. A study in a mouse model has confirmed that bone marrow cells infused into the peripheral circulation do indeed home in on peri-infarct areas [95]. However, the number of cells that reach the affected area is small, and the technique would be most applicable only after an AMI, because it would rely on physiologic homing signals alone. Moreover, since peripherally infused stem cells "home" to infarcted areas only when injected within a few days after an AMI, this delivery strategy would be much less suitable for treating chronic myocardial ischemia.

The major drawback to using an intravenous route of cell delivery would be the possibility that the therapeutic cells would become trapped in the microvasculature of the lungs, liver, and lymphoid tissues. This theoretical limitation of systemic transvenous delivery of stem cells has been confirmed experimentally. In a study by Toma et al. [97], human MSCs were injected into the left ventricular cavity of experimental mice; 4 days later, an estimated 0.44% of the injected cells remained in the myocardium, and the rest had localized to the spleen, liver, and lungs. Other studies using the systemic delivery approach have produced similar results, with very low local cell retention rates of less than 5% [98, 99]. Thus, the transvenous delivery route appears unlikely to achieve the local cell concentration needed to produce a significant therapeutic benefit.

Retrograde Coronary Venous Delivery

Two methodologies have been described for delivering therapeutic agents via the coronary venous system. Low-pressure delivery aims to increase the time that the agent is in contact with the vessels without disrupting the venous endothelium [100–102]. High-pressure delivery aims to create a biological reservoir of product by disrupting the tight endothelial junctions of the venocapillary vasculature and mechanically driving cells across them into the myocardial interstitium [103–105]. Another, newer technique involves a new catheter that has proximal and distal balloons that occlude coronary flow and therefore theoretically allow greater contact between therapeutic cells and the coronary venous system.

The clinical experience with retrograde venous infusion is limited, and several key issues, such as optimal delivery pressure, volume, and infusion time, remain to be resolved.

Intracoronary Infusion

Intracoronary infusion has been the most popular method of delivering stem cells in the clinical setting, especially after AMI. Intracoronary stem cell delivery 4–9 days after AMI is relatively safe [106–112]. The technique is similar to that for coronary angioplasty, which involves over-the-wire positioning of an angioplasty balloon in a coronary artery (Fig. 7.9). Coronary blood flow is transiently stopped for 2–4 min while stem cells are infused under pressure. This maximizes their contact with the microcirculation of the infarct-related artery, thereby optimizing their homing time. Again, this delivery technique would be suitable only in the setting of acute ischemia when adhesion molecules and cytokine signaling are temporarily upregulated.

Results of recent studies have challenged the safety and effectiveness of intracoronary delivery. There is growing evidence of very low retention of stem cells in target regions and of increased restenosis rates associated with this delivery method.

Intramyocardial Injection

Intramyocardial injection has been performed in the clinical setting of chronic myocardial ischemia. It is the preferred delivery route in patients with chronic total occlusion of coronary arteries and in patients with chronic conditions (e.g., congestive heart failure) that involve weaker homing signals. In theory, intramyocardial injection should be the most suitable route for delivering larger cells such as skeletal myoblasts and MSCs, which are prone to microvascular "plugging." Intramyocardial injection can be performed via transepicardial, transendocardial, or transcoronary venous routes.

Transepicardial Injection

Transepicardial injection of stem cells has been performed during open surgical revascularization procedures to deliver the cells to infarct border zones or areas of infarcted or scarred myocardium. Because a sternotomy is required, this approach is highly invasive and associated with surgical complications. However, in the setting of a planned open

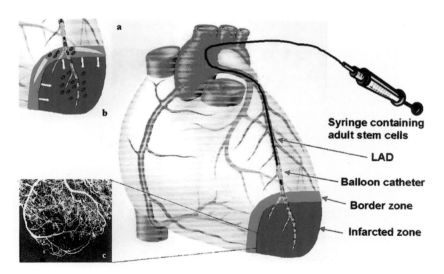

Fig. 7.9 Intracoronary stem cell delivery. The technique is similar to that for coronary angioplasty, which involves over-the-wire positioning of an angioplasty balloon in a coronary artery. Coronary blood flow is transiently stopped for 2–4 min while stem cells are infused under pressure, maximizing their contact with the microcirculation of the infarct-related artery and optimizing their homing time. This delivery technique would be suitable only in the setting of acute ischemia when adhesion molecules and cytokine signaling are temporarily upregulated

heart procedure, the ancillary delivery of cell therapy in this fashion can be easily justified. Interestingly, not all areas of the myocardium (e.g., the interventricular septum) can be reached via a direct external approach.

The main advantages of direct surgical injection are its proven safety in several preclinical and human trials [38, 63, 113–118] and ease of use. However, it is also costly and offers a very unsophisticated targeting opportunity. The surgeon uses visual assessment only to inject the border of the infarcted area or scar tissue. In addition, the safety of direct surgical injection in patients with recent AMI has not been tested in clinical trials. Nevertheless, direct surgical injection might certainly have a role in the future of stem cell therapy. For example, a cardiac surgeon during coronary artery bypass grafting surgery could bypass all areas in which it is technically feasible to do so and then concomitantly inject stem cells into areas of totally occluded epicardial coronary arteries.

Transendocardial Injection

Transendocardial injection is performed via a percutaneous femoral approach. An injection-needle catheter is advanced in retrograde fashion across the aortic valve and positioned against the endocardial surface. Stem cells are then injected directly into targeted areas of the left ventricular wall. Three catheter systems are currently available for transendocardial cell delivery: the Stilleto™ (Boston Scientific, Natick, MA), the BioCardia™ (BioCardia South, San Francisco, CA) (Fig. 7.10), and the Myostar™ (Biosense Webster, Diamond Bar, CA).

The Stilleto is used under fluoroscopic (usually biplanar) guidance. Drawbacks of the approach are the bidimensional orientation and lack of precision associated with fluoroscopy. Another drawback is the inability to characterize the underlying or target myocardium. Nevertheless, this technology may be promising when used with other imaging technologies, such as magnetic resonance imaging (MRI), or when targeting of myocardial therapy is not necessary. Toward this end, in preclinical experiments, the Stilleto catheter has been coupled with real-time cardiac MRI, which permits online assessment of full-thickness myocardium and perfusion. Though still investigational and not currently practical in terms of clinical application, the simultaneous use of MRI offers three-dimensional spatial orientation. Few preclinical studies have been performed, and no safety data from human studies have been assessed [119]. Theoretically, the use of MRI also provides a unique opportunity to track the intramyocardial retention of therapeutic cells after direct injection. This will,

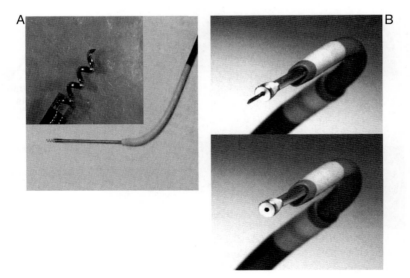

Fig. 7.10 Photos illustrating representative endocardial injection catheters currently under study. Pictured are the helical Biocardia catheter (**A**) and the spring-loaded Boston Scientific Stiletto™ (**B**). Reprinted from [169]

however, require the labeling of cells (specifically MSCs) with fluorescent iron particles that can be detected in the beating heart.

The BioCardia delivery system uses a catheter whose deflectable tip includes a helical needle for infusion. Initial preclinical and clinical experience with this system has provided preliminary evidence of its safety and feasibility [120, 121]. Unlike the other two catheter delivery systems discussed here, the BioCardia catheter does not offer any additional navigational or targeting tool. More extensive preclinical experience with this catheter is needed before future human trials can begin.

The Myostar injection catheter takes advantage of nonfluoroscopic magnetic guidance (Fig. 7.11) [122]. Injections are targeted with the help of a three-dimensional left ventricular "shell," or NOGA electromechanical map (EMM), representing the endocardial surface of the left ventricle. The shell is constructed by acquiring a series of electrocardiogram-gated points at multiple locations on the endocardial surface. Ultralow magnetic fields $(10^-$ to 10^{-6} Tesla) generated by a triangular magnetic pad positioned beneath the patient intersect with a sensor just proximal to the deflectable tip of a 7F mapping catheter, which helps determine the real-time location and orientation of the catheter tip inside the left ventricle. The NOGA system algorithmically calculates and analyzes the

movement of the catheter tip or the location of an endocardial point throughout systole and diastole. That movement is then compared with the movement of neighboring points in an area of interest. The resulting value, called linear local shortening (LLS), is expressed as a percentage that represents the degree of mechanical function of the left ventricular region at that endocardial point. Data are obtained only when the catheter tip is in stable contact with the endocardium. This contact is determined automatically.

The mapping catheter also incorporates electrodes that measure endocardial electrical signals (unipolar or bipolar voltage) [122]. Voltage values are assigned to each point acquired during left ventricular mapping, and an electrical map is constructed concurrently with the mechanical map. Each data point has an LLS value and a voltage value. When the map is complete, all the data points are integrated by the NOGA workstation into a three-dimensional color-coded map of the endocardial surface, as well as 9- and 12-segment bull's-eye views that show average LLS and voltage values in each myocardial segment (Fig. 12). These maps can be spatially manipulated in real time on a Silicon Graphics workstation (Mountain View, CA). The three-dimensional representations acquired during the cardiac cycle can also be used to calculate left ventricular volume and ejection fraction.

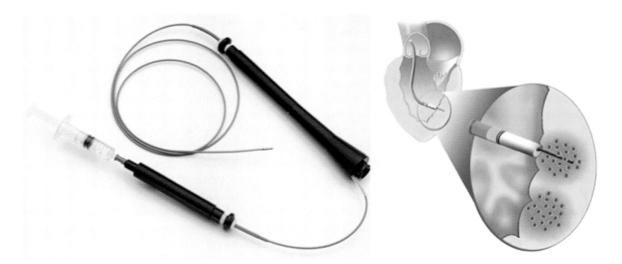

Fig. 7.11 (*Left*) Myostar catheter with attached syringe. (*Right*) Artist's illustration showing the catheter traversing the aortic valve and transendocardial extension of the needle with cell delivery (inset). Reprinted from [26]

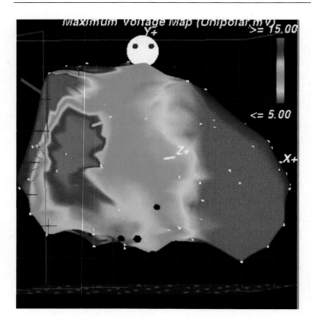

Fig. 7.12 Electromechanical map, in the anterior orientation, depicting unipolar voltage. The red area at the apex of the left ventricle denotes the lowest values and corresponds to scar tissue

The three-dimensional EMM serves both therapeutic and diagnostic purposes. On the one hand, it allows the catheter to be maneuvered through the left ventricle and oriented for transendocardial injections. On the other hand, it allows ischemic areas (i.e., those with low LLS and preserved unipolar voltage [UniV]) to be distinguished from infarcted areas (i.e., those with low LLS and low UniV) [123]. Moreover, the Myostar catheter allows myocardial viability to be assessed at each specific injection site where the catheter touches the endocardial surface. The operator is thus able to target therapy to viable tissue (where neoangiogenesis may be possible) or nonviable tissue (where the target of cell therapy may be a scarred area). Because of the patchy nature of human ischemic heart disease, the ability to characterize the underlying myocardial tissue is important when delivering stem cells.

The EMM technology has been widely tested in both animals and humans and has an excellent safety profile [26, 124–130]. Kornowski et al. [128] have studied the dynamics of transendocardial delivery using different needle extensions to inject 0.1 cc of methylene blue dye as a tracer. A total of 152 injections were performed with needle extensions varying from 3 to 4 mm in length. Two myocardial regions were injected per animal, and injection sites were located after the animals were sacrificed acutely. Staining extended to a depth of 7.1±2.1 mm (range, 2–11 mm) and to a width of 2.3±1.8 mm (range, 1–9 mm). In 2.6% of cases (4 of 152), the injected dye stained the epicardial surface, suggesting pericardial extravasation; more importantly, three of those four injections were made in the apical area. There were no animal deaths, no instances of pericardial effusion or tamponade, and no episodes of sustained ventricular arrhythmia associated with the transendocardial injections.

Despite the limitations of the animal model, this preclinical experience has translated well into clinical trials. However, it is very important to note that the clinical safety profile of transendocardial delivery so far has entailed precise preinjection measurements of needle extension with the injection catheter tip deflected (to 90 degrees) and not deflected, arbitrary insistence on a maximal needle-to-wall ratio of 0.6, and a conscious decision not to inject stem cells into cardiac walls that are less than 8 mm thick or into the true apical segment.

The EMM technology has evolved and now EMMs can be performed in a short period of time using a new platform of NOGA XP (Fig. 7.13).

Transcoronary Venous Injection

Transcoronary venous injection is performed with a catheter system threaded percutaneously into the coronary sinus. Initial studies in swine have confirmed the feasibility and safety of this approach [121]. This delivery method has also been used to deliver skeletal myoblasts to scarred myocardium in cardiomyopathy patients [120]. With intravascular ultrasound guidance, this approach allows the operator to extend a catheter and needle away from the pericardial space and coronary artery into the adjacent myocardium. To date, human feasibility studies have had a good safety profile. This technique is limited, however, by coronary venous tortuosity, lack of site specific targeting, and its own technically challenging nature. Unlike the transendocardial approach, in which cells are

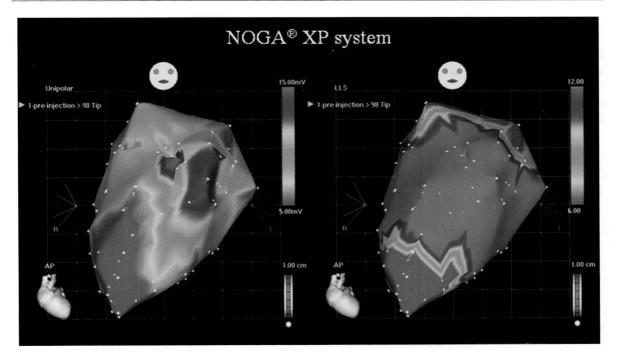

Fig. 7.13 Electromechanical map of the left ventricle performed with the NOGA® XP platform in an acute ovine model of myocardial ischemia (anteroapical myocardial infarction). (*Left*) Unipolar voltage mapping (color scale in mV). (*Right*) Linear local shortening mapping (color scale in %)

injected perpendicularly into the left ventricular wall, the transcoronary venous approach allows parallel cell injection, which may result in greater cell retention.

Comparisons of Delivery Methods

The biodistribution of intravenously injected allogeneic MSCs has been recently described [131]. Oxine-labeled MSCs were injected intravenously 72 h after occlusion/reperfusion in seven dogs. Initially, cells were trapped in the lungs; within 24 h after injection, they had been redistributed into the liver and spleen. Focal uptake and persistence of the stem cells was observed in a mid anterior wall location corresponding to the infarcted target area.

Few studies have compared the different modes of cell delivery. Hou et al. [132] have described the fate of peripheral blood mononuclear cells (PBMNCs) 1 h after direct surgical injection,

intracoronary infusion, and retrograde venous infusion in an acute swine ischemia/reperfusion model. Overall, PBMNCs concentrated significantly more in the pulmonary vasculature and parenchyma than in the myocardium. Direct surgical injection resulted in significantly less pulmonary retention (26%) than did either intracoronary infusion (47%) or retrograde venous infusion (43%). Cells were scarcely present in the liver and spleen. Myocardial homing, even in a setting of intense homing signaling, was limited in all three approaches, although direct intramyocardial injection (11.3%) achieved better homing and engraftment than did either intracoronary infusion (2.6%) or retrograde venous infusion (3.2%).

Together, these data suggest that none of these three delivery strategies are more than modestly efficient at delivering cells to targeted regions. This is of special concern in the case of intracoronary delivery, which is the stem cell delivery method most widely used after AMI. This has several important clinical implications for the future of cardiac stem cell therapy: higher doses might be needed to achieve desired therapeutic effects, new (e.g., combined) delivery strategies need to be considered, myocardial homing and signaling must be better understood, and recipients of systemically delivered cells must be followed up carefully and closely.

Clinical Trials of Cardiac Stem Cell Therapy

Clinical research with bone marrow-derived stem cells has focused on the period immediately after an AMI and on the chronic phase of ischemic heart disease. In these clinical scenarios, therapy has been targeted to viable myocardium with or without systolic heart failure. On the other hand, skeletal myoblast therapy has been used to treat ischemic heart failure involving nonviable myocardium or scar

tissue and compromised systolic left ventricular function. In simple terms, skeletal myoblasts offer "myocyte replacement therapy" for scarred myocardial segments, and bone marrow stem cells offer "neoangiogenic and regenerative therapy" for acute and chronic ischemic heart disease involving viable myocardial tissue.

Most of the clinical experience gained with stem cells has involved therapy for AMI, particularly intracoronary infusion of bone marrow cells since skeletal myoblasts are too large for this purpose [133]. Table 7.2 summarizes the experience to date. In all of these trials, revascularization was performed promptly after the index myocardial infarction, and left ventricular systolic compromise was minor (in the BOOST trial, the baseline left ventricular ejection fraction [LVEF] was 50%).

In the Transplantation of Progenitor Cells and Regeneration Enhancement in Acute Myocardial Infarction (TOPCARE-AMI) trial, patients were randomized to receive either bone marrow-derived

Table 7.2 Trials of intracoronary cell therapy in patients with acute myocardial infarction

Study	[n]	Cell Type	Dose	Time After *AMI*	Therapeutic Effects	
					Improved	No Change
Nonrandomized						
Strauer et al. [111]	10 treated 10 controls*	ABMMNC	$2.8\pm2.2\times10^7$	5–9 days	Regional wall motion† Perfusion† ↓ Infarct size	Global LVEF, LVEDV†
TOPCARE-AMI [106, 107, 110]	29 ABMMNC 30 CPC 11 controls*	ABMMNC, CPC	$2.1\pm0.8\times10^8$ $1.6\pm1.2\times10^7$	5±2 days	Regional wall motion† Global LVEF† ↓ Infarct size† Coronary flow†	LVEDV†
Fernandez-Aviles et al. [109]	20 treated 13 controls*	ABMMNC	$7.8\pm4.1\times10^7$	14±6 days	Regional wall motion† Global LVEF†	LVEDV†
Randomized						
BOOST [112]	30 treated, 30 controls	NC	$2.5\pm0.9\times10^{10}$	6±1 days	Regional wall motion Global LVEF	LVEDV Infarct size
Chen et al. [108]	34 treated 35 controls	MSC	$4.8\pm6.0\times10^{10}$	18 days	Regional wall motion Global LVEF ↓ Infarct size ↓ LVEDV	

* Nonrandomized control groups. †Effects reported only within cell therapy groups. Values are mean ± standard deviation. ABMMNC, autologous bone marrow-derived mononuclear cells; AMI, acute myocardial infarction; BOOST, Bone Marrow Transfer to Enhance ST Elevation Infarct Regeneration; CPC, circulating blood-derived progenitor cells; LVEDV, left ventricular end-diastolic volume; LVEF, left ventricular ejection fraction; MSC, mesenchymal stem cells; NC, bone marrow-derived nucleated cells; TOPCARE, Transplantation of Progenitor Cells and Regeneration Enhancement. Adapted from [170] with permission.

mononuclear cells or EPCs via intracoronary infusion [106]. Compared with the nonrandomized control patients, treated patients had a significantly improved global LVEF, as assessed by left ventricular angiography, regardless of cell type used. In a subgroup of this study population, LVEF was significantly increased, as assessed by cardiac MRI, and infarct size was reduced, as assessed by late-enhancement MRI [107]. Interestingly, the infused cells' ability to migrate was the most important predictor of infarct remodeling. Coronary flow reserve also increased, which is suggestive of neovascularization.

The 1-year results of TOPCARE-AMI reinforce the notion that stem cells protect against ventricular remodeling. Despite the limited number of patients, contrast-enhanced MRI revealed a significantly increased LVEF ($P < 0.001$), significantly reduced infarct size ($P < 0.001$), and the absence of reactive hypertrophy, suggesting that the infarcted ventricles had been functionally regenerated. Scientific criticism of this trial has focused on the cell delivery method, which included transient coronary occlusion and flow cessation, and its potential for ischemic preconditioning. Such preconditioning has been shown to improve outcomes during AMI and may have contributed to the functional improvement noted in this trial. Moreover, the occurrence of in-stent thrombosis in one patient 3 days after undergoing cell therapy has raised safety concerns.

In a study by Bartunek et al. [134], 35 patients were infused with AC133$^+$ bone marrow cells after AMI. The mean dose was 12.6 million cells, and the mean infusion was 11.4 days after the index event. At 4-month follow-up, treated patients had an improved mean LVEF but higher rates of stent restenosis, stent reocclusion, and de novo coronary artery lesions than did the controls.

The intracoronary route has also been used to deliver autologous MSCs. Chen et al. [108] recently reported the first randomized clinical trial of these cells in 69 patients who underwent a primary percutaneous coronary intervention within 12 h after an AMI. Either MSCs or saline was injected into the target coronary artery. At 3-month follow-up, left ventricular perfusion and the LVEF had significantly improved in the treatment group.

In the randomized BOOST trial [112], patients received either bone marrow-derived ABMMNCs or no treatment at all (no placebo). Stem cell therapy resulted in an increased LVEF and a reduced end-systolic volume, as assessed by MRI. This improvement was attributed principally to increased contractility of the peri-infarct zones. Unlike earlier nonrandomized trials, the BOOST trial did not show a significant reduction in infarct size.

The 18-month follow-up of patients in the BOOST trial was recently published [135]. The initial improvement in LVEF in the cell-treated group was not sustained when compared to the control group. However, the speed in which there was LVEF recovery over the 18 months was significantly higher in the cell-treated group.

A study by Janssens et al. [136] sheds further insight into the intracoronary delivery of ABMMNCs after AMI. In a series of 67 patients, ABMMNCs were infused 24 h after mechanical reperfusion. The primary end point of LVEF at 4-month follow-up was similar between the cell treated and placebo groups. However, the cell treated group had smaller infarct sizes and a better recovery in regional systolic function.

Taken together, the phase I intracoronary delivery trials have taught us that the magnitude of improvement after intracoronary infusion of stem cells is modest and possibly mediated through prevention of remodeling. Overall, the small (less than 5%) cell engraftment after intracoronary delivery could potentially explain its modest therapeutic benefits. More specifically, in Janssens' study [136], the importance of cell-delivery timing is once more evident. Early infusion of stem cells may result in even lower engraftment rates or higher rates of cell death given the adverse environment into which the cells are delivered. Alternatively, the modest therapeutic benefit could be due to patient selection. All of the intracoronary studies were performed in patients with small areas of infarction and a preserved LVEF. As mentioned earlier, animal models of cell delivery have repeatedly shown the superior engraftment of cells via intramyocardial delivery.

The feasibility and efficacy of granulocyte-colony stimulating factor (G-CSF) therapy and subsequent intracoronary infusion of collected peripheral blood stem cells were prospectively investigated in the MAGIC randomized clinical trial [137], which showed improved cardiac function and promotion of angiogenesis in myocardial infarction patients.

However, the trial raised important safety questions. Intracoronary infusion of G-CSF-stimulated peripheral-blood stem cells apparently aggravated restenosis after coronary stenting, leading to early termination of the trial. Meanwhile, no temporal association between increased restenosis rate and stenting near the time of intracoronary cell administration has been noted in other studies that have not used G-CSF stimulation.

A different therapeutic strategy using G-CSF involved mobilization of $CD34^+$ cells from the bone marrow to the peripheral blood [32]. Thirty patients in the superacute phase of MI underwent primary percutaneous revascularization. Eighty-five minutes after revascularization, 15 patients were randomized to begin receiving G-CSF stimulation for up to 6 days. At 1-year follow-up, the G-CSF-treated patients had significantly improved LVEF and stable end-diastolic diameters.

The safety of G-CSF stimulation in patients with CAD has been questioned in two recent studies. Hill et al. [138] report the results of administration of 10 mcg/kg/day of G-CSF for 5 days in patients with chronic CAD ($n = 16$). There was no clinical benefit as assessed by exercise stress testing and dobutamine cardiac MRI. Additionally two patients in the G-CSF group developed serious adverse events related to the therapy (one non-ST elevation MI; one MI causing death). Zbinden et al. [139] also tested the efficacy of the same G-CSF dose in patients with chronic CAD ($n = 7$). The invasive endpoint collateral flow index was significantly better in the G-CSF treated patients when compared to the placebo group. However, two patients in the G-CSF treated group developed acute coronary syndrome during treatment.

In a study by Zohlnhofer et al. [140], 56 AMI patients were assigned to receive G-CSF treatment after successful percutaneous coronary intervention. Those patients were compared with 58 patients assigned to receive a placebo. The G-CSF treatment did not influence infarct size, left ventricular function, or coronary restenosis, and G-CSF was not associated with adverse outcomes.

Collectively, the G-CSF trials point to an ineffective therapy after AMI and in the chronic setting that could be potentially dangerous due to systemic inflammatory effects that likely lead to acute coronary syndromes.

Outside the AMI setting, stem cells have been used to treat patients with ischemic heart disease with or without systolic functional compromise and patients unsuitable for myocardial revascularization (Tables 7.3 and 7.4). Autologous bone marrow stem cells have been used to treat patients with chronic myocardial ischemia, including ischemic heart failure with or without systolic functional compromise, and patients ineligible for myocardial revascularization (Table 7.4). The preliminary clinical evidence supports the efficacy of this new therapy and, at this point, all the evidence appears to substantiate its safety.

Tse et al. [130] have reported that transendocardial injection of autologous BMMNCs in eight patients with severe ischemic heart disease led to preserved left ventricular function. At 3-month follow-up, heart failure symptoms and myocardial perfusion had improved, especially in the ischemic region as shown by cardiac MRI.

Fuchs et al. [124] studied the clinical feasibility of transendocardial delivery of filtered unfractionated autologous bone marrow-derived (not mononuclear) cells in ten patients with severe, symptomatic, chronic myocardial ischemia not amenable to conventional revascularization. Twelve targeted injections (0.2 mL each) were administered into ischemic, noninfarcted myocardium identified previously by single-photon emission computed tomography (SPECT) perfusion imaging. No serious adverse effects (i.e., arrhythmia, infection, myocardial inflammation, or increased scar formation) were noted. Moreover, even though treadmill exercise duration results did not change significantly (391 ± 155 versus 485 ± 198 seconds; $P = 0.11$), there was improvement in Canadian Cardiovascular Society angina scores (3.1 ± 0.3 versus 2.0 ± 0.94; $P = 0.001$) and in stress scores in segments within the injected regions (2.1 ± 0.8 versus 1.6 ± 0.8; $P < 0.001$).

Our group performed the first clinical trial of transendocardial injection of ABMMCs to treat heart failure patients [26]. This study, performed in collaboration with physicians and scientists at the Hospital Pro-Cardiaco in Rio de Janeiro, Brazil, used EMM-guided transendocardial delivery of stem cells. The results of 2- and 4-month noninvasive and invasive follow-up evaluations [26] and of 6- and 12-month follow-up evaluation [129] have already been published.

Table 7.3 Cell therapy trials in patients with ischemic cardiomyopathy

Study	[n]	LVEF	Cell Type	Dose	Time After MI	Delivery	Outcomes in Treated Groups
Menasche et al. [115]	10 treated	24±4%	Myoblasts	$8.7±1.9×10^8$	3–228 months	Transepicardial (during CABG)*	↑ Regional wall motion ↑ Global LVEF
Herreros et al. [114]	11 treated	36±8%	Myoblasts	$1.9±1.2×10^8$	3–168 months	Transepicardial (during CABG)†	↑ Regional wall motion ↑ Global LVEF ↑ Viability in infarct area
Siminiak et al. [116]	10 treated	25–40%	Myoblasts	$0.04–5.0×10^7$	4–108 months	Transepicardial (during CABG)†	↑ Regional wall motion ↑ Global LVEF
Chachques et al. [162]	20 treated	28±3%	Myoblasts	$3.0±0.2×10^8$	Not reported	Transepicardial (during CABG)*	↑ Regional wall motion ↑ Global LVEF ↑ Viability in infarct area
Smits et al. [163]	5 treated	36±11%	Myoblasts	$2.0±1.1×10^8$	24–132 months	Transendocardial (guided by EMM)	↑ Regional wall motion ↑ Global LVEF
Stamm et al. [117, 118]	12 treated	36±11%	CD133 +	$1.0–2.8×10^6$	3–12 weeks	Transepicardial (during CABG)*	↑ Global LVEF ↑ Perfusion ↓ LVEDV
Assmus et al. [164]	51 ABMMNC 35 CPC 16 controls	40±11%	ABMMNC CPC	$1.7±0.8×10^8$ $2.3±1.2×10^7$	3–144 months	IC	↑ Global LVEF (only in ABMMNC group)

* CABG of noninjected territories only; †CABG of injected and noninjected territories. Values are mean ± standard deviation. ABMMNC, autologous bone marrow mononuclear cells; AMI, acute myocardial infarction; BM, bone marrow; CABG, coronary artery bypass grafting; CD133 +, bone marrow-derived CD133 + cells; CPC, circulating blood-derived progenitor cells; EMM, electromechanical mapping; IC, intracoronary; LVEDV, left ventricular end-diastolic volume; LVEF, left ventricular ejection fraction; MI, myocardial infarction; NYHA, New York Heart Association. Adapted from [170] with permission.

Table 7.4 Cell therapy trials in patients with myocardial ischemia and no revascularization option

Study	[n]	LVEF	Cell Type	Dose	Delivery	Outcomes Subjective	Objective
Hamano et al. [113]	5 treated	–	ABMMNC	$0.3–2.2×10^9$	Transepicardial (during CABG)	–	↑ Perfusion†
Tse et al. [130]	8 treated	58±11%	ABMMNC	From 40 mL BM	Transendocardial (guided by EMM)	↓ Angina†	↑ Perfusion† ↑ Regional wall motion†
Fuchs et al. [165]	10 treated	47±10%	NC	$7.8±6.6×10^7$	Transendocardial (guided by EMM)	↓ Angina†	↑ Perfusion†
Perin et al. [26, 129]	14 treated 7 controls*	30±6%	ABMMNC	$3.0±0.4×10^7$	Transendocardial (guided by EMM)	↓ Angina ↓ NYHA class	↑ Perfusion ↑ Regional wall motion† ↑ Global LVEF

* Nonrandomized control group; ↑Effects reported only within cell therapy groups. Values are mean ± standard deviation. ABMMNC, autologous bone marrow-derived mononuclear cells; BM, bone marrow; CABG, coronary artery bypass grafting; EMM, electromechanical mapping; LVEF, left ventricular ejection fraction; NC, bone marrow-derived nucleated cells; NYHA, New York Heart Association. Adapted from [170] with permission.

Table 7.5 Comparison of clinical values for the treatment and control groups at baseline, 2, 6, and 12 months

Variable	Baseline		2 Mo		6 Mo		12 Mo		P Value*
	Rx	Control	Rx	Control	Rx	Control	Rx	Control	
SPECT									
Total reversible defect, %	14.8±14.5	20±25.4	4.45±11.5	37±38.4	8.8±9	32.7±37	11.3±12.8	34.3±30.8	0.01
Total fixed defect (50%), %	42.6±10.3	38±12	39.8±6.9	39.1±11.2	38±6.7	36.4±12	38.2±8.5	35.2±9.3	0.3
Ramp Treadmill Test									
VO$_2$ max, mL/kg/min	17.3±8	17.5±6.7	23.2±8	18.3±9.6	24.2±7	17.3±6	25.1±8.7	18.2±6.7	0.03
METS	5.0±2.3	5.0±1.91	6.6±2.3	5.2±2.7	7.2±2.4	4.9±1.7	7.2±2.5	5.1±1.9	0.02
LVEF	30±6	37±14	37±6	27±6	30±10	28±4	35.1±6.9	34±3	0.9
Functional Class									
NYHA	2.2±0.9	2.7±0.8	1.5±0.5	2.4±1.0	1.3±0.6	2.4±0.5	1.4±0.7	2.7±0.5	0.01
CCSAS	2.6±0.8	2.9±1.0	1.8±0.6	2.5±0.8	1.4±0.5	2±0.1	1.2±0.4	2.7±0.5	0.002
PVCs, n	2507±6243	672±1085	901±1236	2034±4528	3902±8267	1041±1971	–	–	0.4
dQRS, ms	136±15	145±61	145.9±25	130±27	144.8±25	140±61	–	–	0.62
LAS 40, ms	50±24	70±76	54±33	48±20	25±25	66±79	–	–	0.47
RMS 40, μv	22.2±22	23.3±23	23.3±19	24.6±28	25±25	30±27	–	–	0.7

*P value for comparisons between the treatment and control groups, as assessed by ANOVA, relating to treatment over time. CCSAS, Canadian Cardiovascular Society Angina Score; dQRS, filtered QRS duration; LAS 40, duration of terminal low-amplitude signal less than 40 mV; LEVF, left ventricular ejection fraction; METS, metabolic equivalents; NYHA, New York Heart Association; PVCs, premature ventricular contractions; RMS 40, root mean square voltage in the terminal 40 ms of the QRS complex; Rx, treatment; SPECT, single-photon emission computer tomography; VO$_2$ max, maximal rate of oxygen consumption. Reprinted from [129] with permission.

Table 7.6 Correlation of bone marrow mononuclear cell subpopulations and reduction in total reversible perfusion defects

Cell population and phenotype	r	P
Hematopoietic progenitor cells (CD45^{lo}CD34$^+$)	0.6	0.04
Early hematopoietic progenitor cells (CD45^{lo}CD34$^+$HLA-DR$^-$)	0.6	0.04
CD4$^+$ T cells (CD45$^+$CD3$^+$CD4$^+$)	0.5	0.1
CD8$^+$ T cells (CD45$^+$CD3$^+$CD8$^+$)	0.5	0.07
B cells (CD45$^+$CD19$^+$)	0.7	0.02
Monocytes (CD45$^+$CD14$^+$)	0.8	0.03
NK cells (CD45$^+$CD56$^+$)	0.1	0.9
B-cell progenitors (CD34$^+$CD19$^+$)	0.5	0.3
CRU-F	0.7	0.06

r indicates Pearson correlation coefficient; CFU-F, fibroblast colony-forming unit; NK, natural killer. Reprinted from [129] with permission.

A total of 21 patients were enrolled. The first 14 comprised the treatment group, and the last 7 patients the control group. Baseline evaluations included complete clinical and laboratory tests, exercise stress (ramp treadmill) studies, two-dimensional Doppler echocardiography, SPECT perfusion scanning, and 24-hour Holter monitoring. ABMMNCs were harvested, isolated, washed, and resuspended in saline for injection via NOGA catheter (15 injections of 0.2 cc, totalling 30×10^6 cells per patient) in viable myocardium (unipolar voltage ≥ 6.9 mV). All patients underwent noninvasive follow-up tests at 2 months, and the treatment group also underwent invasive studies at 4 months, using standard protocols and the same procedures as at baseline. The demographic and exercise test variables did not differ significantly between the treatment and control groups. There were no procedural complications. At 2 months, there was a significant reduction in the total reversible defect in the treatment group and between the treatment and control groups ($P = 0.02$) on quantitative SPECT analysis. At 4 months, the LVEF improved from a baseline of 20 to 29% ($P = 0.003$) and the end-systolic volume decreased ($P = 0.03$) in the treated patients. Electromechanical mapping revealed significant mechanical improvement in the injected segments ($P < 0.0005$). In our opinion, this established the safety of transendocardial injection of ABMMNCs and warranted further investigation of this therapy's efficacy endpoints. This trial was important because for the first time myocardial perfusion and cardiac function were observed to improve in a group of severely impaired patients treated solely with stem cells. The significant improvement seen at 2 and 4 months was maintained at 6 and 12 months, even as exercise capacity improved slightly (Table 7.5). Monocyte, B-cell, hematopoietic progenitor cell, and early hematopoietic progenitor cell subpopulations correlated with improvement in reversible perfusion defects at 6 months (Table 7.6).

Clinical trials of skeletal myoblasts have focused on the treatment of patients with ischemic cardiomyopathy and systolic dysfunction. Overall, these trials have resulted in improved segmental contractility and global LVEF. The preferred delivery route has been surgical intramyocardial injection, and one feasibility trial of transendocardial injection has been reported in the literature so far.

Stem Cell-Induced Functional Improvement in Myocardial Ischemia

Evidence from Preclinical Studies

Preclinical experiments have provided solid evidence supporting the efficacy of cardiac ABMMNC therapy; however, further investigation at the molecular level is needed to elucidate the mechanistic aspects of stem cell therapy—an area where more questions than answers remain.

Numerous research groups, using various detection methods in diverse experimental settings, have proposed different mechanisms for the apparent transformation of stem cells into cells of a variety of tissues [5]. Some investigators attribute the transformation to the transdifferentiation potential of stem cells [141, 142], while others have it to be a result of cell fusion [143].

Initial evidence indicates that ABMMNCs transdifferentiate into endothelial cells and cardiac myocytes. Recent studies in mice, however, have controversially challenged this notion. In a recent study, Murry et al. [144] could detect no ABMMNC transdifferentiation into a cardiomyocyte phenotype, even though sophisticated genetic techniques for following cell fate and engraftment were utilized. However, despite those sophisticated methods of engraftment detection, several critical methodological limitations have been attributed to that study. A study by Kajstura et al. [143] strongly refutes the methodology of Murray's study and describes that c-Kit positive bone marrow cells do transdifferentiate into myocytes as assessed by clear-cut markers of cell identification, such as the presence of Y chromosomes.

In experimental models, ABMMNCs have been shown to depend on external signals that trigger secretory properties and differentiation [145]. The local environment of viable myocardial cells may provide the milieu necessary for inducing ABMMNC myocyte differentiation [146]. In recent studies of occlusion-induced myocardial infarction in rats, few (if any) ABMMNCs might be expected to differentiate and express specific cardiac myocyte proteins, depending on the injection site. To further clarify the issue of transdifferentiation versus fusion, Zhang et al. [147] elegantly used flow cytometry analysis to study heart cell isolates from mice that had received human $CD34^+$ cells. HLA-ABC and cardiac troponin T or Nkx2.5 were used to identify cardiomyocytes derived from human $CD34^+$ cells, and HLA-ABC and VE-cadherin were used to identify the transformed endothelial cells. The double-positive cells were tested for the expression of human and mouse X chromosomes. As a result, 73.3% of nuclei derived from HLA^+ and troponin T^+ or Nkx2.5$^+$ cardiomyocytes contained both human and mouse X chromosomes, and 23.7% contained only human X chromosomes. In contrast, the nuclei of HLA^-, troponin T^+ cells contained only mouse X chromosomes. Furthermore, 97.3% of endothelial cells derived from

$CD34^+$ cells contained human X chromosomes only. Thus, human $CD34^+$ cells both fused with and transdifferentiated into cardiomyocytes in this mouse model. In addition, human $CD34^+$ cells also transdifferentiated into endothelial cells.

The transdifferentiation of HSCs into a mature hematopoietic fate (e.g., endothelium) in the heart is less controversial [148]. In animal models of stem cell therapy in ischemic heart disease, the evidence points toward increased neovascularization (with reduced myocardial ischemia) and consequent improvement in cardiac function [149–151]. Bone marrow stem cells may directly contribute to an increase in contractility or, more likely, may passively limit infarct expansion and remodeling. Unfortunately, the limitations of the present animal models leave this question unanswered.

According to the current understanding of bone marrow stem cell engraftment, most cells die within the first days after delivery. Arteriogenesis and vasculogenesis have long been known to be highly dependent on vascular growth factors. In light of the notion, recently proposed by Kinnaird et al. [133, 152], that MSCs contribute to angiogenesis by means of paracrine mechanisms, it may be that therapeutic bone marrow stem cells recruit circulating progenitor cells, activate resident CSCs, or both, via such paracrine means, thus triggering a cascade of events resulting in cardiac repair. The important role of resident CSCs in the process of cardiac repair should also be considered [82]. Urbanek et al. [37] were the first to describe evidence of myocyte formation from CSCs in human cardiac hypertrophy.

Thum et al. [153] have provided an alternative explanation for the functional improvement seen with stem cell therapy after AMI. They propose that stem cells produce an immunomodulating effect that would, in turn, reduce scar formation, repress cardiac apoptosis, and, thus, improve cardiac function (Fig. 7.14).

Evidence from Clinical Trials

We recently described the postmortem study of one of our patients who received ABMMNCs [154]. Eleven months after performing the treatment, we

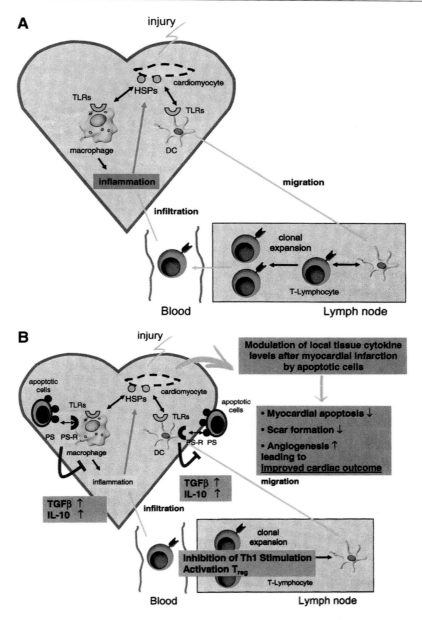

Fig. 7.14 (**A**) Immune pathophysiology of myocardial injury. Ischemic injury damages parenchymal cells, resulting in exposition of heat-shock proteins (HSPs) that trigger tissue-resident macrophages and immature dendritic cells (DCs) via Toll-like receptor 4 (TLR-4) activation. Activated macrophages release several inflammatory cytokines, further amplifying tissue injury, whereas immature DCs undergo maturation and migration to secondary lymphoid tissues. After DC–T-cell interaction, HSP-specific T cells undergo clonal expansion and effector-T-cell differentiation. Homing of these cells to the injured tissue further amplifies local inflammation. (**B**) Apoptotic cells interact with the immune pathophysiology of myocardial injury. Transplanted, ex vivo, induced apoptotic cells or cells undergoing in vivo massive apoptosis inhibit macrophages and DCs via interaction of their surface phosphatidylserine with the respective receptors (PS-R) on the immune cells. As a result, local release of anti-inflammatory cytokines like transforming growth factor (TGF)-beta and interleukin (IL)-10 rises, maturation and migration of DCs and T helper type 1 (Th1) activation is inhibited, and activation of regulatory T cells (Treg) is enhanced. Consequently, less myocardial inflammation is observed, resulting in less myocardial apoptosis and scar formation as well as enhanced angiogenesis. Reprinted from [153]

observed no abnormal or disorganized tissue growth, no abnormal vascular growth, and no enhanced inflammatory reactions. Histologic and immunohistochemical findings from infarcted areas of the anterolateral ventricular wall (areas that had received bone marrow cell injections) compared with findings from within the interventricular septum (which had normal perfusion in the central

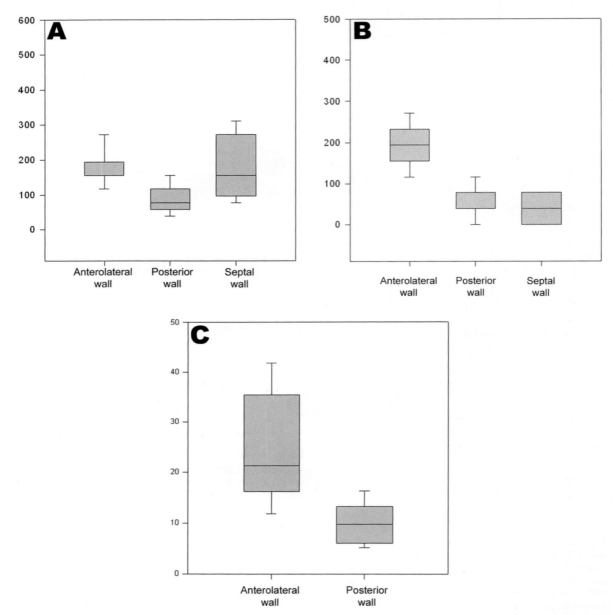

Fig. 7.15 Number of capillaries per mm^2 in anterolateral, posterior, and septal walls of studied heart. (**A**) Anti-factor VIII-associated antigen counterstained with hematoxylin. (**B**) Anti-smooth muscle-actin antigen counterstained with hematoxylin. (**C**) Capillaries reacted with anti-factor VIII-associated antigen inside fibrotic areas only in anterolateral and posterior walls. (*n* = 108 microscope fields for **A**; 96 microscope fields for **B**; and 40 microscope fields for **C**.) Differences were statistically significant among all groups in pair-wise comparisons (*P* < 0.05, Newman-Keuls method) for **A** and **B**. Differences were significantly different (*P* < 0.05) between anterolateral and posterior walls in Mann-Whitney rank-sum test for **C**. Reprinted from [154]

region and no cell therapy) and from the previously infarcted inferoposterior ventricular wall (which had extensive scarring and no cell therapy).

The observed effects of cell therapy in this one patient were intriguing: first, the cell-treated infarcted areas of this patient's heart had a higher capillary density than did the nontreated, infarcted areas (Fig. 7.15). Second, smooth muscle α-actin-positive pericytes and mural cells proliferated exclusively in the cell-treated area. Third, these pericytes and mural cells expressed specific cardiomyocyte proteins.

The angiogenesis literature makes clear that pericytes are essential for long-lasting physiological angiogenesis. In our postmortem study, the cell-injected wall had marked areas of pericyte and mural cells hyperplasia. The observed hypertrophic pericytes, though still located in the vascular wall, expressed specific myocardial proteins and were found in locations distant from the vessel walls, suggesting detachment. Migratory pericytes and mural cells were found in adjacent tissue (in the vicinity of cardiomyocytes) either isolated or in small clumps. Closer to cardiomyocytes, the expression of myocardial proteins was enhanced, yielding brighter immunostaining throughout the whole cytoplasm. Within the posterior wall, none of this was seen, and small blood vessels were rare. Although it would be premature to arrive at any definitive conclusions about ABMMNC efficacy on the basis of one postmortem study, the above findings in the cell-treated wall are consistent with neoangiogenesis. If confirmed in future human studies, these findings would corroborate earlier findings from most of the preclinical studies in chronic myocardial ischemia models.

Safety of Stem Cell Therapy

With regard to left ventricular function, cardiac stem cell therapy is well tolerated overall. No proarrhythmic effects have been observed to date with ABMMNC therapy, although other deleterious effects are possible. Early concerns about abnormal transdifferentiation and tumorigenesis have subsided, but the potential for accelerated atherogenesis remains, given the limited clinical experience

and the small number of patients treated. Because atherosclerosis is an inflammatory disease triggered and sustained by cytokines, adhesion molecules, and cellular components such as monocytes and macrophages, intracoronary delivery is potentially risky. In addition, as already mentioned, post-MI intracoronary infusion has been associated with increased rates of restenosis and stent thrombosis. Given the small number of patients treated in all phase I/II trials so far, this is a particular point of concern.

Another potential deleterious effect of bone marrow stem cell therapy is myocardial calcification. In a recent study, Yoon et al. [155] noted that direct transplantation of unselected bone marrow cells into acutely infarcted myocardium could induce significant intramyocardial calcification. In the same study, however, ABMMNCs did not.

Myoblast therapy raises the possibility of arrhythmogenic effects. Consequently, many clinical studies require the placement of cardiac defibrillators in patients receiving myoblasts.

Conclusions

Despite many unresolved issues related to treatment dose, timing, and delivery, the clinical potential of stem cell therapy for cardiovascular disease is enormous. The expectations of both patients and clinicians for this new therapeutic modality, however, are high and to achieve the full potential stem cell therapy has to offer will require continued cooperation and future close collaboration between basic and clinical scientists.

References

1. Radovancevic B, Vrtovec B, Frazier OH. Left ventricular assist devices: an alternative to medical therapy for end-stage heart failure. *Curr Opin Cardiol* 2003;18:210–214.
2. Asahara T, Murohara T, Sullivan A, Silver M, van der Zee R, Li T, Witzenbichler B, Schatteman G, Isner JM. Isolation of putative progenitor endothelial cells for angiogenesis. *Science* 1997;275:964–967.
3. Shintani S, Murohara T, Ikeda H, Ueno T, Honma T, Katoh A, Sasaki K, Shimada T, Oike Y, Imaizumi T.

Mobilization of endothelial progenitor cells in patients with acute myocardial infarction. *Circulation* 2001;103:2776–2779.

4. Krause DS. Plasticity of marrow-derived stem cells. *Gene Ther* 2002;9:754–758.

5. Perin EC, Geng YJ, Willerson JT. Adult stem cell therapy in perspective. *Circulation* 2003;107:935–938.

6. Blau HM, Brazelton TR, Weimann JM. The evolving concept of a stem cell: entity or function? *Cell* 2001;105:829–841.

7. Weissman IL. Stem cells: units of development, units of regeneration, and units in evolution. *Cell* 2000;100: 157–168.

8. www.nih.org; accessed May 22, 2006.

9. Korbling M, Estrov Z. Adult stem cells for tissue repair – a new therapeutic concept? *N Engl J Med* 2003;349: 570–582.

10. Rumpold H, Wolf D, Koeck R, Gunsilius E. Endothelial progenitor cells: a source for therapeutic vasculogenesis? *J Cell Mol Med* 2004;8:509–518.

11. Asahara T, Masuda H, Takahashi T, Kalka C, Pastore C, Silver M, Kearne M, Magner M, Isner JM. Bone marrow origin of endothelial progenitor cells responsible for postnatal vasculogenesis in physiological and pathological neovascularization. *Circ Res* 1999;85:221–228.

12. Asahara T, Takahashi T, Masuda H, Kalka C, Chen D, Iwaguro H, Inai Y, Silver M, Isner JM. VEGF contributes to postnatal neovascularization by mobilizing bone marrow-derived endothelial progenitor cells. *EMBO J* 1999;18:3964–3972.

13. Bhattacharya V, McSweeney PA, Shi Q, Bruno B, Ishida A, Nash R, Storb RF, Sauvage LR, Hammond WP, Wu MH. Enhanced endothelialization and microvessel formation in polyester grafts seeded with CD34(+) bone marrow cells. *Blood* 2000;95:581–585.

14. Edelberg JM, Tang L, Hattori K, Lydon D, Rafii S. Young adult bone marrow-derived endothelial precursor cells restore aging-impaired cardiac angiogenic function. *Circ Res* 2002;90:E89–93.

15. Gehling UM, Ergun S, Schumacher U, Wagener C, Pantel K, Otte M, Schuch G, Schafhausen P, Mende T, Kilic N, Kluge K, Schafer B, Hossfeld DK, Fiedler W. In vitro differentiation of endothelial cells from AC133-positive progenitor cells. *Blood* 2000;95:3106–3112.

16. Gill M, Dias S, Hattori K, River ML, Hicklin D, Witte L, Girardi L, Yurt R, Himel H, Rafii S. Vascular trauma induces rapid but transient mobilization of VEGFR2(+)AC133(+) endothelial precursor cells. *Circ Res* 2001;88:167–174.

17. Gunsilius E, Petzer AL, Duba HC, Kahler CM, Gastl G. Circulating endothelial cells after transplantation. *Lancet* 2001;357:1449–1450.

18. Hatzopoulos AK, Folkman J, Vasile E, Eiselen GK, Rosenberg RD. Isolation and characterization of endothelial progenitor cells from mouse embryos. *Development* 1998;125:1457–1468.

19. Iwaguro H, Yamaguchi J, Kalka C, Murasawa S, Masuda H, Hayashi S, Silver M, Li T, Isner JM, Asahara T. Endothelial progenitor cell vascular endothelial growth factor gene transfer for vascular regeneration. *Circulation* 2002;105:732–738.

20. Kalka C, Masuda H, Takahashi T, Kalka-Moll WM, Silver M, Kearney M, Li T, Isner JM, Asahara T. Transplantation of ex vivo expanded endothelial progenitor cells for therapeutic neovascularization. *Proc Natl Acad Sci U S A* 2000;97:3422–3427.

21. Kaushal S, Amiel GE, Guleserian KJ, Shapira OM, Perry T, Sutherland FW, Rabkin E, Moran AM, Schoen FJ, Atala A, Soker S, Bischoff J, Mayer JE Jr. Functional small-diameter neovessels created using endothelial progenitor cells expanded ex vivo. *Nat Med* 2001;7: 1035–1040.

22. Lin Y, Weisdorf DJ, Solovey A, Hebbel RP. Origins of circulating endothelial cells and endothelial outgrowth from blood. *J Clin Invest* 2000;105:71–77.

23. Murohara T, Ikeda H, Duan J, Shintani S, Sasaki K, Eguchi H, Onitsuka I, Matsui K, Imaizumi T. Transplanted cord blood-derived endothelial precursor cells augment postnatal neovascularization. *J Clin Invest* 2000;105:1527–1536.

24. Nieda M, Nicol A, Denning-Kendall P, Sweetenham J, Bradley B, Hows J. Endothelial cell precursors are normal components of human umbilical cord blood. *Br J Haematol* 1997;98:775–777.

25. Peichev M, Naiyer AJ, Pereira D, Zhu Z, Lane WJ, Williams M, Oz MC, Hicklin DJ, Witte L, Moore MA, Rafii S. Expression of VEGFR-2 and AC133 by circulating human CD34(+) cells identifies a population of functional endothelial precursors. *Blood* 2000;95: 952–958.

26. Perin EC, Dohmann HF, Borojevic R, Silva SA, Sousa AL, Mesquita CT, Rossi MI, Carvalho AC, Dutra HS, Dohmann HJ, Silva GV, Belem L, Vivacqua R, Rangel FO, Esporcatte R, Geng YJ, Vaughn WK, Assad JA, Mesquita ET, Willerson JT. Transendocardial, autologous bone marrow cell transplantation for severe, chronic ischemic heart failure. *Circulation* 2003;107: 2294–2302.

27. Schatteman GC, Hanlon HD, Jiao C, Dodds SG, Christy BA. Blood-derived angioblasts accelerate blood-flow restoration in diabetic mice. *J Clin Invest* 2000;106:571–578.

28. Shi Q, Rafii S, Wu MH, Wijelath ES, Yu C, Ishida A, Fujita Y, Kothari S, Mohle R, Sauvage LR, Moore MA, Storb RF, Hammond WP. Evidence for circulating bone marrow-derived endothelial cells. *Blood* 1998;92: 362–367.

29. Springer ML, Chen AS, Kraft PE, Bednarski M, Blau HM. VEGF gene delivery to muscle: potential role for vasculogenesis in adults. *Mol Cell* 1998;2:549–558.

30. Takahashi T, Kalka C, Masuda H, Chen D, Silver M, Kearney M, Magner M, Isner JM, Asahara T. Ischemia- and cytokine-induced mobilization of bone marrow-derived endothelial progenitor cells for neovascularization. *Nat Med* 1999;5:434–438.

31. Vasa M, Fichtlscherer S, Aicher A, Adler K, Urbich C, Martin H, Zeiher AM, Dimmeler S. Number and migratory activity of circulating endothelial progenitor cells inversely correlate with risk factors for coronary artery disease. *Circ Res* 2001;89:E1–7.

32. Iwami Y, Masuda H, Asahara T. Endothelial progenitor cells: past, state of the art, and future. *J Cell Mol Med* 2004;8:488–497.

33. Ferrari G, Cusella-De Angelis G, Coletta M, Paolucci E, Stornaiuolo A, Cossu G, Mavilio F. Muscle regeneration by bone marrow-derived myogenic progenitors. *Science* 1998;279:1528–1530.

34. Graf T. Differentiation plasticity of hematopoietic cells. *Blood* 2002;99:3089–3101.

35. Beltrami AP, Barlucchi L, Torella D, Baker M, Limana F, Chimenti S, Kasahara H, Rota M, Musso E, Urbanek K, Leri A, Kajstura J, Nadal-Ginard D, Anversa P. Adult cardiac stem cells are multipotent and support myocardial regeneration. *Cell* 2003;114:763–776.

36. Oh H, Bradfute SB, Gallardo TD, Nakamura T, Gaussin V, Mishina Y, Pocius J, Michael LH, Behringer RR, Garry DJ, Entman ML, Schneider MD. Cardiac progenitor cells from adult myocardium: homing, differentiation, and fusion after infarction. *Proc Natl Acad Sci U S A* 2003;100:12313–12318.

37. Urbanek K, Quaini F, Tasca G, Torella D, Castaldo C, Nadal-Ginard D, Leri A, Kajstura J, Quaini E, Anversa P. Intense myocyte formation from cardiac stem cells in human cardiac hypertrophy. *Proc Natl Acad Sci U S A* 2003;100:10440–10445.

38. Orlic D, Kajstura J, Chimenti S, Jakoniuk I, Anderson SM, Li B, Pickel J, McKay R, Nadal-Ginard B, Bodine DM, Leri A, Anversa P. Bone marrow cells regenerate infarcted myocardium. *Nature* 2001;410:701–705.

39. Quaini F, Urbanek K, Beltrami AP, Finato N, Beltrami CA, Nadal-Ginard B, Kajstura J, Leri A, Anversa P. Chimerism of the transplanted heart. *N Engl J Med* 2002;346:5–15.

40. Kucia M, Ratajczak J, Ratajczak MZ. Bone marrow as a source of circulating CXCR4+ tissue-committed stem cells. *Biol Cell* 2005;97:133–146.

41. Rafii S, Lyden D. Therapeutic stem and progenitor cell transplantation for organ vascularization and regeneration. *Nat Med* 2003;9:702–712.

42. Fadini GP, Miorin M, Facco M, Bonamico S, Baesso I, Grego F, Menegolo M, de Kreutzenberg SV, Tiengo A, Agostini C, Avogaro A. Circulating endothelial progenitor cells are reduced in peripheral vascular complications of type 2 diabetes mellitus. *J Am Coll Cardiol* 2005;45:1449–1457.

43. Walter DH, Haendeler J, Reinhold J, Rochwalsky U, Seeger F, Honold J, Urbich C, Lehmann R, Arezana-Seisdesdos F, Aicher A, Heeschen C, Fichtlscherer S, Zeiher AM, Dimmeler S. Impaired CXCR4 signaling contributes to the reduced neovascularization capacity of endothelial progenitor cells from patients with coronary artery disease. *Circ Res* 2005;97:1142–1151.

44. Dong C, Crawford LE, Goldschmidt-Clermont PJ. Endothelial progenitor obsolescence and atherosclerotic inflammation. *J Am Coll Cardiol* 2005;45:1458–1460.

45. Werner N, Kosiol S, Schiegl T, Ahlers P, Walenta K, Link A, Bohm M, Nickenig G. Circulating endothelial progenitor cells and cardiovascular outcomes. *N Engl J Med* 2005;353:999–1007.

46. Schmidt-Lucke C, Rossig L, Fichtlscherer S, Vasa M, Britten M, Kamper U, Dimmeler S, Zeiher AM. Reduced number of circulating endothelial progenitor cells predicts future cardiovascular events: proof of concept for the clinical importance of endogenous vascular repair. *Circulation* 2005;111:2981–2987.

47. Baksh D, Song L, Tuan RS. Adult mesenchymal stem cells: characterization, differentiation, and application in cell and gene therapy. *J Cell Mol Med* 2004;8:301–316.

48. Bruder SP, Jaiswal N, Haynesworth SE. Growth kinetics, self-renewal, and the osteogenic potential of purified human mesenchymal stem cells during extensive subcultivation and following cryopreservation. *J Cell Biochem* 1997;64:278–294.

49. Bruder SP, Kurth AA, Shea M, Hayes WC, Jaiswal N, Kadiyala S. Bone regeneration by implantation of purified, culture-expanded human mesenchymal stem cells. *J Orthop Res* 1998;16:155–162.

50. Kadiyala S, Young RG, Thiede MA, Bruder SP. Culture expanded canine mesenchymal stem cells possess osteochondrogenic potential in vivo and in vitro. *Cell Transplant* 1997;6:125–134.

51. Awad HA, Butler DL, Boivin GP, Smith FN, Malaviya P, Huibregtse B, Caplan AI. Autologous mesenchymal stem cell-mediated repair of tendon. *Tissue Eng* 1999;5:267–277.

52. Young RG, Butler DL, Weber W, Caplan AI, Gordon SL, Fink DJ. Use of mesenchymal stem cells in a collagen matrix for Achilles tendon repair. *J Orthop Res* 1998;16:406–413.

53. Galmiche MC, Koteliansky VE, Briere J, Herve P, Charbord P. Stromal cells from human long-term marrow cultures are mesenchymal cells that differentiate following a vascular smooth muscle differentiation pathway. *Blood* 1993;82:66–76.

54. Dennis JE, Merriam A, Awadallah A, Yoo JU, Johnstone B, Caplan AI. A quadripotential mesenchymal progenitor cell isolated from the marrow of an adult mouse. *J Bone Miner Res* 1999;14:700–709.

55. Prockop DJ. Marrow stromal cells as stem cells for non-hematopoietic tissues. *Science* 1997;276:71–74.

56. Barry FP. Mesenchymal stem cell therapy in joint disease. *Novartis Found Symp* 2003;249:86–96; discussion 96–102, 170–104, 239–141.

57. Chapel A, Bertho JM, Bensidhoum M, Fouillard L, Young RG, Frick J, Demarquay C, Cuvelier F, Mathieu E, Trompier F, Dudoignon N, Germain C, Mazurier C, Aigueperse J, Borneman J, Gorin NC, Gourmelon P, Thierry D. Mesenchymal stem cells home to injured tissues when co-infused with hematopoietic cells to treat a radiation-induced multi-organ failure syndrome. *J Gene Med* 2003;5:1028–1038.

58. Deng Y, Guo X, Yuan Q, Li S. Efficiency of adenoviral vector mediated CTLA4Ig gene delivery into mesenchymal stem cells. *Chin Med J (Engl)* 2003;116:1649–1654.

59. Ortiz LA, Gambelli F, McBride C, Gaupp D, Baddoo M, Kaminski N, Phinney DG. Mesenchymal stem cell engraftment in lung is enhanced in response to bleomycin exposure and ameliorates its fibrotic effects. *Proc Natl Acad Sci U S A* 2003;100:8407–8411.

60. Saito T, Kuang JQ, Bittira B, Al-Khaldi A, Chiu RC. Xenotransplant cardiac chimera: immune tolerance of adult stem cells. *Ann Thorac Surg* 2002;74:19–24; discussion 24.

61. Pittenger MF, Martin BJ. Mesenchymal stem cells and their potential as cardiac therapeutics. *Circ Res* 2004;95:9–20.

62. Tse WT, Pendleton JD, Beyer WM, Egalka MC, Guinan EC. Suppression of allogeneic T-cell proliferation by human marrow stromal cells: implications in transplantation. *Transplantation*2003;75:389–397.

63. Silva GV, Litovsky S, Assad JA, Sousa AL, Martin BJ, Vela D, Coulter SC, Lin J, Ober J, Vaughn WK, Branco RV, Oliveira EM, He R, Geng YJ, Willerson JT, Perin EC. Mesenchymal stem cells differentiate into an endothelial phenotype, enhance vascular density, and improve heart function in a canine chronic ischemia model. *Circulation* 2005;111:150–156.

64. Mangi AA, Noiseux N, Kong D, He H, Rezvani M, Ingwall JS, Dzau VJ. Mesenchymal stem cells modified with Akt prevent remodeling and restore performance of infarcted hearts. *Nat Med*2003;9:1195–1201.

65. Tang YL, Tang Y, Zhang YC, Qian K, Shen L, Phillips MI. Improved graft mesenchymal stem cell survival in ischemic heart with a hypoxia-regulated heme oxygenase-1 vector. *J Am Coll Cardiol* 2005;46:1339–1350.

66. Quirici N, Soligo D, Caneva L, Servida F, Bossolasco P, Deliliers GL. Differentiation and expansion of endothelial cells from human bone marrow CD133(+) cells. *Br J Haematol* 2001;115:186–194.

67. Thomson JA, Itskovitz-Eldor J, Shapiro SS, Waknitz MA, Swiergiel JJ, Marshall VS, Jones JM. Embryonic stem cell lines derived from human blastocysts. *Science* 1998;282:1145–1147.

68. Hristov M, Erl W, Weber PC. Endothelial progenitor cells: mobilization, differentiation, and homing. *Arterioscler Thromb Vasc Biol* 2003;23:1185–1189.

69. Harraz M, Jiao C, Hanlon HD, Hartley RS, Schatteman GC. CD34- blood-derived human endothelial cell progenitors. *Stem Cells*2001;19:304–312.

70. Yoon CH, Hur J, Park KW, Kim JH, Lee CS, Oh IY, Kim TY, Cho HJ, Kang HJ, Chae IH, Yang HK, Oh BH, Park YB, Kim HS. Synergistic neovascularization by mixed transplantation of early endothelial progenitor cells and late outgrowth endothelial cells: the role of angiogenic cytokines and matrix metalloproteinases. *Circulation* 2005;112:1618–1627.

71. Kucia M, Dawn B, Hunt G, Guo Y, Wysoczynski M, Majka M, Ratajczak J, Rezzoug F, Ildstad ST, Bolli R, Ratajczak MZ. Cells expressing early cardiac markers reside in the bone marrow and are mobilized into the peripheral blood after myocardial infarction. *Circ Res* 2004;95:1191–1199.

72. Deb A, Wang S, Skelding KA, Miller D, Simper D, Caplice NM. Bone marrow-derived cardiomyocytes are present in adult human heart: A study of gender-mismatched bone marrow transplantation patients. *Circulation* 2003;107:1247–1249.

73. Dowell JD, Rubart M, Pasumarthi KB, Soonpaa MH, Field LJ. Myocyte and myogenic stem cell transplantation in the heart. *Cardiovasc Res* 2003;58:336–350.

74. Menasche P. Cellular transplantation: hurdles remaining before widespread clinical use. *Curr Opin Cardiol* 2004;19:154–161.

75. Leor J, Patterson M, Quinones MJ, Kedes LH, Kloner RA. Transplantation of fetal myocardial tissue into the infarcted myocardium of rat. A potential method for repair of infarcted myocardium? *Circulation* 1996;94(9 Suppl):II332–336.

76. Tambara K, Sakakibara Y, Sakaguchi G, Lu F, Premaratne GU, Lin X, Nishimura K, Komeda M. Transplanted skeletal myoblasts can fully replace the infarcted myocardium when they survive in the host in large numbers. *Circulation* 2003;108 Suppl 1:II259–263.

77. Williams RL, Hilton DJ, Pease S, Wilson TA, Stewart CL, Gearing DP, Wagner EF, Metcalf D, Nicola NA, Gough NM. Myeloid leukaemia inhibitory factor maintains the developmental potential of embryonic stem cells. *Nature* 1988;336:684–687.

78. Cowan CA, Klimanskaya I, McMahon J, Atienza J, Witmyer J, Zucker JP, Wang S, Morton CC, McMahon AP, Powers D, Melton DA. Derivation of embryonic stem-cell lines from human blastocysts. *N Engl J Med* 2004;350:1353–1356.

79. Itskovitz-Eldor J, Schuldiner M, Karsenti D, Eden A, Yanuka O, Amit M, Soreq H, Benvenisty N. Differentiation of human embryonic stem cells into embryoid bodies compromising the three embryonic germ layers. *Mol Med* 2000;6:88–95.

80. Sachinidis A, Fleischmann BK, Kolossov E, Wartenberg M, Sauer H, Hescheler J. Cardiac specific differentiation of mouse embryonic stem cells. *Cardiovasc Res* 2003;58:278–291.

81. Lovell MJ, Mathur A. The role of stem cells for treatment of cardiovascular disease. *Cell Prolif* 2004;37:67–87.

82. Anversa P, Sussman MA, Bolli R. Molecular genetic advances in cardiovascular medicine: focus on the myocyte. *Circulation* 2004;109:2832–2838.

83. Urbanek K, Rota M, Cascapera S, Bearzi C, Nascimbene A, De Angelis A, Hosoda T, Chimenti S, Baker M, Limana F, Nurzynska D, Torella D, Rotatori F, Rastaldo R, Musso E, Quaini F, Leri A, Kajstura J, Anversa P. Cardiac stem cells possess growth factor-receptor systems that after activation regenerate the infarcted myocardium, improving ventricular function and long-term survival. *Circ Res* 2005;97:663–673.

84. Messina E, De Angelis L, Frati G, Morrone S, Chimenti S, Fiordaliso F, Salio M, Battaglia M, Latronico MV, Coletta M, Vivarelli E, Frati L, Cossu G, Giacomello A. Isolation and expansion of adult cardiac stem cells from human and murine heart. *Circ Res* 2004;95:911–921.

85. Dragoo JL, Choi JY, Lieberman JR, Huang J, Zuk PA, Zhang J, Hedrick MH, Ben haim P. Bone induction by BMP-2 transduced stem cells derived from human fat. *J Orthop Res* 2003;21:622–629.

86. Safford KM, Hicok KC, Safford SD, Halvorsen YD, Wilkison WO, Gimble JM, Rice HE. Neurogenic differentiation of murine and human adipose-derived stromal cells. *Biochem Biophys Res Commun* 2002;294:371–379.

87. Zuk PA, Zhu M, Ashjian P, De Ugarte DA, Huang JI, Mizuno H, Alfonso ZC, Fraser JK, Benhaim P, Hedrick MH. Human adipose tissue is a source of multipotent stem cells. *Mol Biol Cell* 2002;13: 4279–4295.

88. Rehman J, Traktuev D, Li J, Merfeld-Clauss S, Temm-Grove CJ, Bovenkerk JE, Pell CL, Johnstone BH, Considine RV, March KL. Secretion of angiogenic and antiapoptotic factors by human adipose stromal cells. *Circulation* 2004;109:1292–1298.
89. Gronthos S, Franklin DM, Leddy HA, Robey PG, Stroms RW, Gimble JM. Surface protein characterization of human adipose tissue-derived stromal cells. *J Cell Physiol* 2001;189:54–63.
90. Wulf GG, Viereck V, Hemmerlein B, Haase D, Vehmeyer K, Pukrop T, Glass B, Emons G, Trumper L. Mesengenic progenitor cells derived from human placenta. *Tissue Eng* 2004;10:1136–1147.
91. Erices A, Conget P, Minguell JJ. Mesenchymal progenitor cells in human umbilical cord blood. *Br J Haematol* 2000;109:235–242.
92. Jaiswal RK, Jaiswal N, Bruder SP, Mbalaviele G, Marshak DR, Pittenger MF. Adult human mesenchymal stem cell differentiation to the osteogenic or adipogenic lineage is regulated by mitogen-activated protein kinase. *J Biol Chem* 2000;275:9645–9652.
93. Sims DE. Diversity within pericytes. *Clin Exp Pharmacol Physiol* 2000;27:842–846.
94. Zuk PA, Zhu M, Mizuno H, Huang J, Futrell JW, Katz AJ, Benhaim P, Lorenz HP, Hedrick MH. Multilineage cells from human adipose tissue: implications for cell-based therapies. *Tissue Eng* 2001;7:211–228.
95. Lew WY. Mobilizing cells to the injured myocardium: a novel rescue strategy or an unwelcome intrusion? *J Am Coll Cardiol* 2004;44:1521–1522.
96. Maekawa Y, Anzai T, Yoshikawa T, Sugano Y, Mahara K, Kohno T, Takahashi T, Ogawa S. Effect of granulocyte-macrophage colony-stimulating factor inducer on left ventricular remodeling after acute myocardial infarction. *J Am Coll Cardiol* 2004;44:1510–1520.
97. Toma C, Pittenger MF, Cahill KS, Byrne BJ, Kessler PD. Human mesenchymal stem cells differentiate to a cardiomyocyte phenotype in the adult murine heart. *Circulation* 2002;105:93–98.
98. Aicher A, Brenner W, Zuhayra M, Badorff C, Massoudi S, Assmus B, Eckey T, Henze E, Zeiher AM, Dimmeler S. Assessment of the tissue distribution of transplanted human endothelial progenitor cells by radioactive labeling. *Circulation* 2003;107:2134–2139.
99. Barbash IM, Chouraqui P, Baron J, Feinberg MS, Etzion S, Tessone A, Miller R, Guetta E, Zipori D, Kedes LH, Kloner RA, Leor J. Systemic delivery of bone marrow-derived mesenchymal stem cells to the infarcted myocardium: feasibility, cell migration, and body distribution. *Circulation* 2003;108:863–868.
100. Boekstegers P, von Degenfeld G, Giehrl W, Heinrich D, Hullin R, Kupatt C, Steinbeck G, Baretton G, Middeler G, Katus H, Franz WM. Myocardial gene transfer by selective pressure-regulated retroinfusion of coronary veins. *Gene Ther* 2000;7:232–240.
101. Murad-Netto S, Moura R, Romeo LJ, Manoel Neto A, Duarte N, Barreto F, Jensen A, Vina RF, Vraslovik F, Oberdan A, Benetti F, Saslavsky J, Vina MF, Amino JG. Stem cell therapy with retrograde coronary perfusion in acute myocardial infarction. A new technique. *Arq Bras Cardiol* 2004;83:352–354; 349–351.
102. von Degenfeld G, Raake P, Kupatt C, Lebherz C, Hinkel R, Gildehaus FJ, Munzing W, Kranz A, Waltenberger J, Simoes M, Schwaiger M, Thein E, Boekstegers P. Selective pressure-regulated retroinfusion of fibroblast growth factor-2 into the coronary vein enhances regional myocardial blood flow and function in pigs with chronic myocardial ischemia. *J Am Coll Cardiol* 2003;42:1120–1128.
103. Herity NA, Lo ST, Oei F, Lee DP, Ward MR, Filardo SD, Hassan A, Suzuki T, Rezaee M, Carter AJ, Yock PG, Yeung AC, Fitzgerald PJ. Selective regional myocardial infiltration by the percutaneous coronary venous route: A novel technique for local drug delivery. *Catheter Cardiovasc Interv* 2000;51:358–363.
104. Hou D, Maclaughlin F, Thiesse M, Panchal VR, Bekkers BC, Wilson EA, Rogers PI, Coleman MC, March KL. Widespread regional myocardial transfection by plasmid encoding Del-1 following retrograde coronary venous delivery. *Catheter Cardiovasc Interv* 2003;58:207–211.
105. Raake P, von Degenfeld G, Hinkel R, Vachenauer R, Sandner T, Beller S, Andrees M, Kupatt C, Schuler G, Boekstegers P. Myocardial gene transfer by selective pressure-regulated retroinfusion of coronary veins: comparison with surgical and percutaneous intramyocardial gene delivery. *J Am Coll Cardiol* 2004;44:1124–1129.
106. Assmus B, Schachinger V, Teupe C, Britten M, Lehmann R, Dobert N, Grunwald F, Aicher A, Urbich C, Martin H, Hoelzer D, Dimmeler S, Zeiher AM. Transplantation of Progenitor Cells and Regeneration Enhancement in Acute Myocardial Infarction (TOPCARE-AMI). *Circulation* 2002;106:3009–3017.
107. Britten MB, Abolmaali ND, Assmus B, Lehmann R, Honold J, Schmitt J, Vogl TJ, Martin H, Schachinger V, Dimmeler S, Zeiher AM. Infarct remodeling after intracoronary progenitor cell treatment in patients with acute myocardial infarction (TOPCARE-AMI): mechanistic insights from serial contrast-enhanced magnetic resonance imaging. *Circulation* 2003;108:2212–2218.
108. Chen SL, Fang WW, Ye F, Liu YH, Qian J, Shan SJ, Zhang JJ, Chunhua RZ, Liao LM, Lin S, Sun JP. Effect on left ventricular function of intracoronary transplantation of autologous bone marrow mesenchymal stem cell in patients with acute myocardial infarction. *Am J Cardiol* 2004;94:92–95.
109. Fernandez-Aviles F, San Roman JA, Garcia-Frade J, Fernandez ME, Penarrubia MJ, de la Fuente L, Gomez-Bueno M, Cantalapiedra A, Fernandez J, Gutierrez O, Sanchez PL, Hernandez C, Sanz R, Garcia-Sancho J, Sanchez A. Experimental and clinical regenerative capability of human bone marrow cells after myocardial infarction. *Circ Res* 2004;95:742–748.
110. Schachinger V, Assmus B, Britten MB, Honold J, Lehmann R, Teupe C, Abolmaali ND, Vogl TJ, Hofmann WK, Martin H, Dimmeler S, Zeiher AM. Transplantation of progenitor cells and regeneration enhancement in acute myocardial infarction: final one-year results of the TOPCARE-AMI Trial. *J Am Coll Cardiol* 2004;44:1690–1699.

111. Strauer BE, Brehm M, Zeus T, Kostering M, Hernandez A, Sorg RV, Kogler G, Wernet P. Repair of infarcted myocardium by autologous intracoronary mononuclear bone marrow cell transplantation in humans. *Circulation* 2002;106:1913–1918.

112. Wollert KC, Meyer GP, Lotz J, Ringes-Lichtenberg S, Lippolt P, Breidenbach C, Fichtner S, Korte T, Hornig B, Messinger D, Arseniev L, Hertenstein B, Ganser A, Drexler H. Intracoronary autologous bone-marrow cell transfer after myocardial infarction: the BOOST randomised controlled clinical trial. *Lancet* 2004;364:141–148.

113. Hamano K, Nishida M, Hirata K, Mikamo A, Li TS, Harada M, Miura T, Matsuzaki M, Esato K. Local implantation of autologous bone marrow cells for therapeutic angiogenesis in patients with ischemic heart disease: clinical trial and preliminary results. *Jpn Circ J* 2001;65:845–847.

114. Herreros J, Prosper F, Perez A, Gavira JJ, Garcia-Velloso MJ, Barba J, Sanchez PL, Canizo C, Rabago G, Marti-Climent JM, Hernandez M, Lopez-Holgado N, Gonzalez-Santos JM, Martin-Luengo C, Alegria E. Autologous intramyocardial injection of cultured skeletal muscle-derived stem cells in patients with non-acute myocardial infarction. *Eur Heart J* 2003;24:2012–2020.

115. Menasche P, Hagege AA, Vilquin JT, Desnos M, Abergel E, Pouzet B, Bel A, Sarateanu S, Scorsin N, Schwartz K, Bruneval P, Benbunan M, Marolleau JP, Duboc D. Autologous skeletal myoblast transplantation for severe postinfarction left ventricular dysfunction. *J Am Coll Cardiol* 2003;41:1078–1083.

116. Siminiak T, Kalawski R, Fiszer D, Jerzykowska O, Rzezniczak J, Rozwadowska N, Kurpisz M. Autologous skeletal myoblast transplantation for the treatment of postinfarction myocardial injury: phase I clinical study with 12 months of follow-up. *Am Heart J* 2004;148:531–537.

117. Stamm C, Kleine HD, Westphal B, Petzsch M, Kittner C, Nienaber CA, Freund M, Steinhoff G. CABG and bone marrow stem cell transplantation after myocardial infarction. *Thorac Cardiovasc Surg* 2004;52: 152–158.

118. Stamm C, Westphal B, Kleine HD, Petzsch M, Kittner C, Klinge H, Schumichen C, Nienaber CA, Freund M, Steinhoff G. Autologous bone-marrow stem-cell transplantation for myocardial regeneration. *Lancet* 2003;361:45–46.

119. Hill JM, Dick AJ, Raman VK, Thompson RB, Yu ZX, Hinds KA, Pessanha BS, Guttman MA, Varney TR, Martin BJ, Dunbar CE, McVeigh ER, Lederman RJ. Serial cardiac magnetic resonance imaging of injected mesenchymal stem cells. *Circulation* 2003;108: 1009–1014.

120. Siminiak T, Fiszer D, Jerzykowska O, Grygielska B, Rozwadowska N, Kalmucki P, Kurpisz M. Percutaneous trans-coronary-venous transplantation of autologous skeletal myoblasts in the treatment of post-infarction myocardial contractility impairment: the POZNAN trial. *Eur Heart J* 2005;26:1188–1195.

121. Thompson CA, Nasseri BA, Makower J, Houser S, McGarry M, Lamson T, Pomerantseva I, Chang JY, Gold HK, Vacanti JP, Oesterle SN. Percutaneous transvenous cellular cardiomyoplasty. A novel nonsurgical approach for myocardial cell transplantation. *J Am Coll Cardiol* 2003;41:1964–1971.

122. Sarmento-Leite R, Silva GV, Dohman HF, Rocha RM, Dohman HJ, de Mattos ND, Carvalho LA, Gottechall CA, Perin EC. Comparison of left ventricular electromechanical mapping and left ventricular angiography: defining practical standards for analysis of NOGA maps. *Tex Heart Inst J* 2003;30:19–26.

123. Perin EC, Silva GV, Sarmento-Leite R, Sousa AL, Howell M, Muthupillai R, Lambert B, Vaughn WK, Flamm SD. Assessing myocardial viability and infarct transmurality with left ventricular electromechanical mapping in patients with stable coronary artery disease: validation by delayed-enhancement magnetic resonance imaging. *Circulation* 2002;106:957–961.

124. Fuchs S, Baffour R, Zhou YF, Shou M, Pierre A, Tio FO, Weissman NJ, Leon MB, Epstein SB, Kornowski R. Transendocardial delivery of autologous bone marrow enhances collateral perfusion and regional function in pigs with chronic experimental myocardial ischemia. *J Am Coll Cardiol* 2001;37:1726–1732.

125. Kamihata H, Matsubara H, Nishiue T, Fujiyama S, Amano K, Iba O, Imada T, Iwasaka T. Improvement of collateral perfusion and regional function by implantation of peripheral blood mononuclear cells into ischemic hibernating myocardium. *Arterioscler Thromb Vasc Biol* 2002;22:1804–1810.

126. Kawamoto A, Tkebuchava T, Yamaguchi J, Nishimura H, Yoon YS, Milliken C, Uchida S, Masuo O, Iwaguro H, Ma H, Hanley A, Silver M, Kearney M, Losordo DW, Isner JM, Asahara T. Intramyocardial transplantation of autologous endothelial progenitor cells for therapeutic neovascularization of myocardial ischemia. *Circulation* 2003;107:461–468.

127. Kornowski R, Fuchs S, Tio FO, Pierre A, Epstein SE, Leon MB. Evaluation of the acute and chronic safety of the biosense injection catheter system in porcine hearts. *Catheter Cardiovasc Interv* 1999;48:447–453; discussion 454–445.

128. Kornowski R, Leon MB, Fuchs S, Vodovotz Y, Flynn MA, Gordon DA, Pierre A, Kovesdi I, Keiser JA, Epstein SA. Electromagnetic guidance for catheter-based transendocardial injection: a platform for intramyocardial angiogenesis therapy. Results in normal and ischemic porcine models. *J Am Coll Cardiol* 2000;35:1031–1039.

129. Perin EC, Dohmann HF, Borojevic R, Silva SA, Sousa AL, Silva GV, Mesquita CT, Belem L, Vaughn WK, Rangel FO, Assad JA, Carvalho AC, Branco RV, Rossi MI, Dohmann HJ, Willerson JT. Improved exercise capacity and ischemia 6 and 12 months after transendocardial injection of autologous bone marrow mononuclear cells for ischemic cardiomyopathy. *Circulation* 2004;110(11 Suppl 1):II213–218.

130. Tse HF, Kwong YL, Chan JK, Lo G, Ho CL, Lau CP. Angiogenesis in ischaemic myocardium by intramyocardial autologous bone marrow mononuclear cell implantation. *Lancet* 2003;361:47–49.

131. Kraitchman DL, Tatsumi M, Gilson WD, Ishimori T, Kedziorek D, Walczak P, Segars WP, Chen HH, Fritzges D, Izbudak I, Young RG, Marcelino M, Pittenger MF, Solaiyappan M, Boston RC, Tsui BM, Wahl RL, Bulte JW. Dynamic imaging of allogeneic mesenchymal stem cells trafficking to myocardial infarction. *Circulation* 2005;112:1451–1461.
132. Hou D, Youssef EA, Brinton TJ, Zhang P, Rogers P, Price ET, Yeung AC, Johnstone BH, Yock PG, March KL. Radiolabeled cell distribution after intramyocardial, intracoronary, and interstitial retrograde coronary venous delivery: implications for current clinical trials. *Circulation* 2005;112(9 Suppl):I150–156.
133. Kinnaird T, Stabile E, Burnett MS, Shou M, Lee CW, Barr S, Fuchs S, Epstein SE. Local delivery of marrow-derived stromal cells augments collateral perfusion through paracrine mechanisms. *Circulation* 2004;109:1543–1549.
134. Bartunek J, Vanderheyden M, Vandekerckhove B, Mansour S, De Bruyne B, De Bondt P, Van Haute I, Lootens N, Heyndrickx G, Wijns W. Intracoronary injection of CD133-positive enriched bone marrow progenitor cells promotes cardiac recovery after recent myocardial infarction: feasibility and safety. *Circulation* 2005;112(9 Suppl):I178–183.
135. Meyer GP, Wollert KC, Lotz J, Steffens J, Lippolt P, Fichtner S, Heckner H, Schaefer A, Arseniev L, Hertenstein B, Ganser A, Drexler H. Intracoronary bone marrow cell transfer after myocardial infarction: eighteen months' follow-up data from the randomized, controlled BOOST (BOne marrOw transfer to enhance ST-elevation infarct regeneration) trial. *Circulation* 2006;113:1287–1294.
136. Janssens S, Dubois C, Bogaert J, Theunissen K, Deroose C, Desmet W, Kalantzi M, Herbots L, Sinnaeve P, Dens J, Maertens J, Rademakers F, Dymarkowski S, Gheysens O, Van Cleemput A, Bormans G, Nuyts J, Belmans A, Mortelmans L, Boogaerts M, Van de Werf F. Autologous bone marrow-derived stem-cell transfer in patients with ST-segment elevation myocardial infarction: double-blind, randomised controlled trial. *Lancet* 2006;367:113–121.
137. Kang HJ, Kim HS, Zhang SY, Park KW, Cho HJ, Koo BK, Kim YJ, Soo Lee D, Soon DW, Han KS, Oh BH, Lee MM, Park YB. Effects of intracoronary infusion of peripheral blood stem-cells mobilised with granulocyte-colony stimulating factor on left ventricular systolic function and restenosis after coronary stenting in myocardial infarction: the MAGIC cell randomised clinical trial. *Lancet* 2004;363:751–756.
138. Hill JM, Syed MA, Arai AE, Powell TM, Paul JD, Zalos G, Read EJ, Khuu HM, Leitman SF, Horne M, Csako G, Dunbar CE, Waclawiw MA, Cannon RO 3rd. Outcomes and risks of granulocyte colony-stimulating factor in patients with coronary artery disease. *J Am Coll Cardiol* 2005;46:1643–1648.
139. Zbinden S, Zbinden R, Meier P, Windecker S, Seiler C. Safety and efficacy of subcutaneous-only granulocyte-macrophage colony-stimulating factor for collateral growth promotion in patients with coronary artery disease. *J Am Coll Cardiol* 2005;46:1636–1642.
140. Zohlnhofer D, Ott I, Mehilli J, Schomig K, Michalk F, Ibrahim T, Meisetschlager G, von Wedel J, Bollwein H, Seyfarth M, Dirschinger J, Schmitt C, Schwaiger M, Kastrati A, Schomig A. Stem cell mobilization by granulocyte colony-stimulating factor in patients with acute myocardial infarction: a randomized controlled trial. *JAMA* 2006;295:1003–1010.
141. Goodell MA. Stem-cell "plasticity": befuddled by the muddle. *Curr Opin Hematol* 2003;10:208–213.
142. Hocht-Zeisberg E, Kahnert H, Guan K, Wulf G, Hemmerlein B, Schlott T, Tenderich G, Korfer R, Raute-Kreisen, Hasenfuss G. Cellular repopulation of myocardial infarction in patients with sex-mismatched heart transplantation. *Eur Heart J* 2004;25:749–758.
143. Kajstura J, Rota M, Whang B, Cascapera S, Hosoda T, Bearzi C, Nurzynska D, Kasahara H, Zias E, Bonafe N, Nadal-Ginard B, Torella D, Nascimbene A, Quaini F, Urbanek K, Leri A, Anvera P. Bone marrow cells differentiate in cardiac cell lineages after infarction independently of cell fusion. *Circ Res* 2005;96:127–137.
144. Murry CE, Soonpaa MH, Reinecke H, Nakajima H, Nakajima HO, Rubart M, Pasumarthi KB, Virag JI, Bartelmez SH, Poppa V, Bradford G, Dowell JD, Williams DA, Field LJ. Haematopoietic stem cells do not transdifferentiate into cardiac myocytes in myocardial infarcts. *Nature* 2004;428:664–668.
145. Losordo DW, Dimmeler S. Therapeutic angiogenesis and vasculogenesis for ischemic disease: part II: cell-based therapies. *Circulation* 2004;109:2692–2697.
146. Yeh ET, Zhang S, Wu HD, Korbling M, Willerson JT, Estrov Z. Transdifferentiation of human peripheral blood CD34+-enriched cell population into cardiomyocytes, endothelial cells, and smooth muscle cells in vivo. *Circulation* 2003;108:2070–2073.
147. Zhang S, Wang D, Estrov Z, Raj S, Willerson JT, Yeh ET. Both cell fusion and transdifferentiation account for the transformation of human peripheral blood CD34-positive cells into cardiomyocytes in vivo. *Circulation* 2004;110:3803–3807.
148. Forrester JS, Price MJ, Makkar RR. Stem cell repair of infarcted myocardium: an overview for clinicians. *Circulation* 2003;108:1139–1145.
149. Duan HF, Wu CT, Wu DL, Lu Y, Liu HJ, Ha XQ, Zhang QW, Wang H, Jia XX, Wang LS. Treatment of myocardial ischemia with bone marrow-derived mesenchymal stem cells overexpressing hepatocyte growth factor. *Mol Ther* 2003;8:467–474.
150. Kudo M, Wang Y, Wani MA, Xu M, Ayub A, Ashraf M. Implantation of bone marrow stem cells reduces the infarction and fibrosis in ischemic mouse heart. *J Mol Cell Cardiol* 2003;35:1113–1119.
151. Tang YL, Zhao Q, Zhang YC, Cheng L, Liu M, Shi J, Yang YZ, Pan C, Ge J, Phillips MI. Autologous mesenchymal stem cell transplantation induce VEGF and neovascularization in ischemic myocardium. *Regul Pept* 2004;117:3–10.
152. Kinnaird T, Stabile E, Burnett MS, Lee CW, Barr S, Fuchs S, Epstein SE. Marrow-derived stromal cells express genes encoding a broad spectrum of

arteriogenic cytokines and promote in vitro and in vivo arteriogenesis through paracrine mechanisms. *Circ Res* 2004;94:678–685.

153. Thum T, Bauersachs J, Poole-Wilson PA, Volk HD, Anker SD. The dying stem cell hypothesis: immune modulation as a novel mechanism for progenitor cell therapy in cardiac muscle. *J Am Coll Cardiol* 2005;46:1799–1802.

154. Dohmann HF, Perin EC, Takiya CM, Silva GV, Silva SA, Sousa AL, Mesquita CT, Rossi MI, Pascarelli BM, Assis IM, Dutra HS, Assad JA, Castello-Branco RV, Drummond C, Dohmann HJ, Willerson JT, Borojevic R. Transendocardial autologous bone marrow mononuclear cell injection in ischemic heart failure: postmortem anatomicopathologic and immunohistochemical findings. *Circulation* 2005;112:521–526.

155. Yoon YS, Park JS, Tkebuchava T, Luedeman C, Losordo DW. Unexpected severe calcification after transplantation of bone marrow cells in acute myocardial infarction. *Circulation* 2004;109:3154–3157.

156. Strehlow K, Werner N, Berweiler J, Link A, Dirnagl U, Priller J, Laufs K, Ghaeni L, Milosevic M, Bohm M, Nickenig G. Estrogen increases bone marrow-derived endothelial progenitor cell production and diminishes neointima formation. *Circulation* 2003;107:3059–3065.

157. Adams V, Lenk K, Linke A, Lenz D, Erbs S, Sandri M, Tarnok A, Gielen S, Emmrich F, Schuler G, Hambrecht R. Increase of circulating endothelial progenitor cells in patients with coronary artery disease after exercise-induced ischemia. *Arterioscler Thromb Vasc Biol* 2004;24:684–690.

158. Valgimigli M, Rigolin GM, Fucili A, Porta MD, Soukhomovskaia O, Malagutti P, Bugli AM, Bragotti LZ, Francolini G, Mauro E, Castoldi G, Ferrari R. CD34+ and endothelial progenitor cells in patients with various degrees of congestive heart failure. *Circulation* 2004;110:1209–1212.

159. George J, Herz I, Goldstein E, Abashidze S, Deutch V, Finkelstein A, Michowitz Y, Miller H, Keren G. Number and adhesive properties of circulating endothelial progenitor cells in patients with in-stent restenosis. *Arterioscler Thromb Vasc Biol* 2003;23:e57–60.

160. Dimmeler S, Aicher A, Vasa M, Mildner-Rihm C, Adler K, Tiemann M, Rutten H, Fichtlscherer S, Martin H, Zeiher AM. HMG-CoA reductase inhibitors (statins) increase endothelial progenitor cells via the PI 3-kinase/Akt pathway. *J Clin Invest* 2001;108:391–397.

161. Bahlmann FH, De Groot K, Spandau JM, Landry AL, Hertel B, Duckert T, Boehm SM, Menne J, Haller H, Fliser D. Erythropoietin regulates endothelial progenitor cells. *Blood* 2004;103:921–926.

162. Chachques JC, Herreros J, Trainini J, Juffe A, Rendal E, Prosper F, Genovese J. Autologous human serum for cell culture avoids the implantation of cardioverter-defibrillators in cellular cardiomyoplasty. *Int J Cardiol* 2004;95 Suppl 1:S29–33.

163. Smits PC, van Geuns RJ, Poldermans D, Bountioukos M, Onderwater EE, Lee CH, Maat AP, Serruys PW. Catheter-based intramyocardial injection of autologous skeletal myoblasts as a primary treatment of ischemic heart failure: clinical experience with six-month follow-up. *J Am Coll Cardiol* 2003;42:2063–2069.

164. Assmus B, Honold J, Lehmann R, Pistorius K, Hoffmann WK, Martin H, Schachinger V, Zeiher AM. Transcoronary transplantation of progenitor cells and recovery of left ventricular function in patients with chronic ischemic heart disease: results of a randomized controlled trial. *Circulation* 2004; 110(Suppl III):238.

165. Fuchs S, Satler LF, Kornowski R, Okubagzi P, Weisz G, Baffour R, Waksman R, Weissman NJ, Cerqueira M, Leon MB, Epstein SE. Catheter-based autologous bone marrow myocardial injection in no-option patients with advanced coronary artery disease: a feasibility study. *J Am Coll Cardiol* 2003;41:1721–1724.

166. Chunming Dong, Lawrence E. Crawford, and Pascal J. Goldschmidt-Clermont. Endothelial Progenitor Obsolescence and Atherosclerotic Inflammation. *J Am Coll Cardiol* 2005;45;1458–1460.

167. Mihail Hristov, Christian Weber. Endothelial progenitor cells: characterization, pathophysiology, and possible clinical relevance. *J Cell Mol Med* 2004;8:498–508.

168. Piero Anversa, Jan Kajstura, Annarosa Leri, Roberto Bolli. Life and death of cardiac stem cells: a paradigm shift in cardiac biology. *Circulation* 2006;113:1451–1463.

169. J. M. Zimmet and J. M. Hare. Emerging Role For Bone Marrow Derived Mesenchymal Stem Cells In Myocardial Regenerative Therapy. *Basic Res Cardiol* 2005;100:471–481.

170. Wollert KC, Drexler H. Clinical applications of stem cells for the heart. *Circ Res* 2005;96:151–163.

Chapter 8
The Future of Treatment of Advanced Ischemic Heart Disease

New Technologies and Strategies Being Studied and Their Potential Impact on the Disease

John L. Jefferies, Marianne Bergheim, and Reynolds Delgado

Prediction is very difficult, especially about the future

Niels Bohr

Heart failure continues to be a significant burden on society with a reported prevalence of ~5 million persons in the United States [1]. It will only continue to worsen as our population ages with an estimated prevalence of 10 million by the year 2037. From 1950 to 2000 there was an improvement in the survival rate after the onset of heart failure of 12% per decade ($P = 0.01$ for men and $P = 0.02$ for women) [2]. This indicates that the number of people living with advanced ischemic heart disease and heart failure is growing and they are living with more comorbidities. Improvement in the medical and surgical management of ischemic heart failure has been made over the past few decades but more aggressive strategies will continue to be in demand with the broadening scope of this disease. The heart failure population is shifting over time with a larger percentage of cases due to ischemic heart disease. In recent trials, as much as 70% of outpatients with heart failure have ischemic heart disease as the underlying cause.

Beginning in 2005, the proportion of the US population that is eligible for Medicare benefits has begun to rise and is projected to do so for many years. (Source: HCFA National Health Expenditures Projections 2000–2010. U.S.

Census Data 2000.) The reasons for the rise in heart failure and advanced 'ischemic heart disease are as follows: (1) better treatment of coronary artery disease, (2) survival of acute myocardial infarction, (3) the aging of the population, (4) wider use of implanted defibrillators to prevent sudden death, (5) better medical management, and (6) longer survival of the population in general. Advances are taking place in many areas of science that are making their way into the treatment of heart disease. Exciting advances are occurring in immunology, biochemistry, genetics, nanotechnology, tissue growth, electronic sensors, and device design. As these technologies move forward, we will see more novel approaches in the treatment of advanced ischemic heart disease.

This final chapter will spotlight some of these areas of research and the potential that they hold. In the future we may be able to grow new hearts to replace damaged ones and monitor ischemia and the progression of the disease via the internet and apply new therapies to arrest adverse remodeling before it leads to the syndrome of heart failure. Most of what will be described here is in the realm of research and application to humans in clinical trials is yet to occur. Despite this, these wonderful advances offer hope to patients for the future.

Future treatments for advanced ischemic heart disease may include techniques and technologies which can

J.L. Jefferies (✉)
Texas Heart Institute, St. Luke's Episcopal Hospital, Houston, TX, USA
e-mail: jjefrries@sleh.com

R. Delgado, H.S. Arora (eds.), *Interventional Treatment of Advanced Ischemic Heart Disease*,
DOI 10.1007/978-1-84800-395-8_8, © Springer-Verlag London Limited 2009

- prevent or diagnose ischemic disease before irreversible remodeling occurs,
- revascularize ischemic myocardium in ways that cannot be currently done,
- restore function to infarcted myocardium via replacement of non-functional myocardium or the entire heart,
- mechanically support the failing or ischemic heart without surgery,
- better utilize existing technologies to slow or prevent the progression of the disease, and
- detect and monitor established heart failure or ischemia.

Prevention or Diagnosis of Ischemic Disease Before Irreversible Remodeling Occurs

How Do We Prevent Myocardial Infarction?

Acute myocardial infarction is the most frequent presentation of coronary disease. In patients with known disease, we have tools to predict who will have an infarction but this ability is limited. The future will see advances that will allow us to predict with a high degree of accuracy the risk of MI and which lesions are likely to be causative and in what time frame. Serum markers are not yet widely used as they do not have enough predictive power to prompt expensive or invasive diagnostic procedures. Screening with imaging procedures is expensive and may lead to unnecessary invasive procedures. New technologies are needed to give a level of confidence to justify invasive investigation. Approaches at studying unique new aspects of the electrocardiogram are being investigated. Investigators at NASA are studying high frequency signals (150–250 Hz) in the QRS wave of the electrocardiogram as a tool to screen populations with cardiac disease. It has been documented that 12-lead high frequency (HF) QRS ECG analysis is inexpensive and reproducible [3]. Also, HF ECG may be more accurate than conventional ECG for detecting coronary artery disease and cardiomyopathy [4] (Fig. 8.1A and B). Further studies will be required

to assess the practical uses of this technology but this may allow for much earlier detection of ischemic disease in broader clinical situations.

In patients with known disease, we currently use degree of stenosis as the primary guide to revascularization, however, it has been know for some time that non-critical lesions may be the real culprit in many patients. A more scientific view has involved attempts to characterize the plaque itself to determine need for therapy. With advances in microminiaturization, devices are being developed to do this in vivo. One such strategy uses a tiny ultrasound probe placed in the coronary artery, which analyzes data which may give insight into the makeup of the plaque itself and thus its risk of rupture. Volcano Inc (Ranch Cordova, CA) has made strides in this (Fig. 8.2A and B) and in wires that can measure flow and pressure changes across a stenosis. In the future, such devices may provide data in addition to angiographic appearance which may guide revascularization decisions or changes in medical therapy.

The human genome is becoming more and more appreciated as a significant source to gain insight into ischemic heart disease [5]. There are approximately 26,000 genes encoding for roughly 100,000 proteins. (The proteins outnumber the number of genes due to alternate splicing.) However, technology currently available (although at considerable cost) can generate profiles of health for *individual* patients as well as entire populations. As this becomes more widely available, a shift in the management of heart disease will occur from acute management to prospective preventative care based on unique personal profiles. This will allow for powerful screening opportunities as well as the possibility for early application of gene therapy. Genome wide sequencing has been performed by multiple groups in an attempt to determine a linkage between coronary artery disease and a specific genetic locus. The results thus far have been limited [6–12]. However, pedigree rich genome-wide sequencing has provided potential insight into at least one cause of autosomal dominant inheritance of coronary artery disease. A haplotype on chromosome 15 encoding for a transcription factor was found in a large family to be present in those members affected with coronary disease and absent from those unaffected [13].

The concept of a "final common pathway" for both acquired and inherited cardiomyopathy has

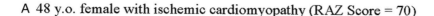

A 48 y.o. female with ischemic cardiomyopathy (RAZ Score = 70)

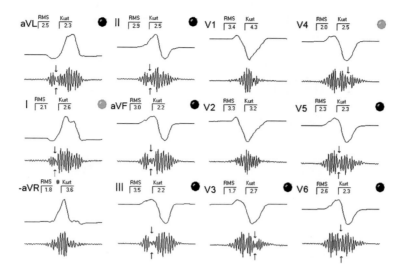

B 49 y.o. female healthy control subject (RAZ Score = 5)

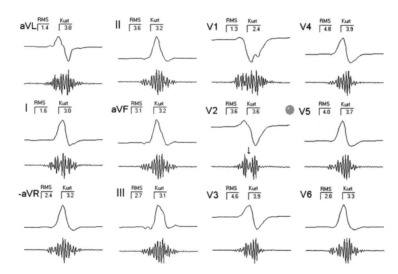

Fig. 8.1 Examples of 12 lead high frequency QRS electrocardiograms from a patient with ischemic cardiomyopathy (**A**) and an age and gender matched healthy control (**B**)

been suggested as a target for further research [14]. Disruptions in the dystrophin gene are a well-recognized cause of cardiomyopathy. Dystrophin is a structural protein that provides support for the myocyte and cardiomyocyte sarcolemmal membrane. Mutations in the dystrophin protein or the dystrophin-associated protein complexes result in skeletal cardiomyopathies [15]. In both dilated and ischemic cardiomyopathy, Vatta et al. demonstrated that both forms were deficient in the N-terminal portion of dystrophin. Furthermore, the amino terminus deficient disease was partially reversible with the use of left ventricular assist devices as demonstrated by immunohistochemical staining [16, 17]. A similar mechanism has been demonstrated in enterovirally induced cardiomyopathy [18]. Specific exon

Fig. 8.2 (**A**) Intravascular ultrasound (IVUS) image of a coronary artery using Revolution 45 MHz IVUS imaging catheter. (**B**) Plaque composition imaging using volcano VH™IVUS system. *Green* areas represent Fibrous plaque. *Yellow* is fibro-fatty areas. *Red* is the necrotic core and white represents areas of dense calcium

A

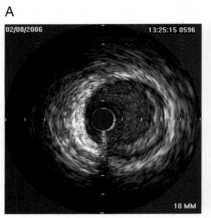

B

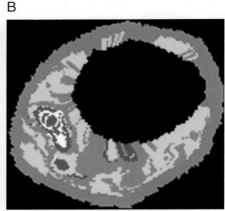

deletions have been implicated in patients with muscular dystrophy, a disease secondary to mutations in the dystrophin gene, as being causative or protective of the onset of dilated cardiomyopathy [19]. If the final common pathway exists, the evaluation of this model may provide insight into the cellular mechanisms of myocyte dysfunction.

The future use of genetics as a practical and affordable screening tool and possible treatment modality is still a few years away. However, technology is advancing rapidly in this field. There is evidence that genetic inflammatory markers, specifically polymorphisms in four genes that are thought to be involved in the inflammatory reaction, may be associated with the need for target vessel revascularization following percutaneous intervention [20]. This may represent a significant finding in patients with ischemic cardiomyopathy as restenosis remains the major limitation to percutaneous revascularization. A major limitation in the past has been the rapidity of base sequencing. This process has been modified allowing for a vast reduction in the time required to assess specific genes. Ultimately, genetic markers associated with cardiac disease will be identified across the entire genome making this a valuable screening tool.

Prevention of heart failure through identification and management of risk factors in the preclinical phase of the disease is a priority. The concept of primary prevention has significant impact on the development of heart failure. It is estimated that the risk factors of hypertension, myocardial infarction, and diabetes contribute to ~80% of the heart failure diagnosed in the United States [21]. More

aggressive screening and treatment could ameliorate a significant portion of the burden heart failure places on society. Primary prevention can only occur if the risk factors are clearly defined and acted upon by the health-care community as well as policy-makers.

Future studies will continue to develop novel and prognostic predictors of heart failure. Protocols for preventing illnesses such as influenza and other infections in patients with advanced heart disease have not become a standard of treatment, but must be emphasized to avoid the worsened outcomes in these "avoidable" situations. Educating the lay-public as well as health-care professionals must be funded and promoted. Numerous studies have documented the inefficiency of prescribing drug therapy that has documented impacts on outcomes in heart failure and coronary artery disease. The utilization of future modalities will not have significant impact without the proper use of established modalities. This may best be accomplished via physicians with a special interest in the area of heart failure. Recent recommendations for the training of heart failure specialists may facilitate this process as well as training physicians to deliver recommended invasive therapies such as cardiac resynchronization in a more effective manner [22].

Greater efforts must be employed to increase the awareness of heart failure in the public eye, specifically the financial burden that it entails as well as the significant morbidity and mortality associated with the diagnosis. Optimization of accepted treatments must be explored on larger scales in patients with ischemic disease and made more widely and affordably available. The tertiary prevention in patients with heart failure may be the area that is the most exciting but also the most distant into the future as outlined above. The most recent AHA/ACC guidelines for the evaluation and management of heart failure address many of these points to a greater degree than previous statements [1]. Wider usage of the guidelines as a conduit to disseminate information to heath care professionals could make significant impacts on heart failure management. Many of the patients that may develop or currently have ischemic heart disease are evaluated and treated by primary care physicians. The education and participation of this group of physicians is critical to a long-term impact on morbidity and mortality.

Revascularize Ischemic Myocardium in Ways that Cannot Currently Be Done

Revascularization remains a critical component in the treatment of ischemic heart disease. Procedures that are currently utilized to revascularize the myocardium include coronary artery bypass grafting (CABG), percutaneous transluminal coronary angioplasty (PTCA) and stenting, and transmyocardial laser revascularization. New methods of surgical revascularization with synthetic grafts and "off-pump" anastamosis devices are being developed to target patients who lack healthy native vessels to harvest or those who are considered high risk for use of the heart lung machine. As discussed in this text, patients who are poor surgical candidates due to comorbidities have received benefit from the use of novel circulatory support systems to avoid hemodynamic complications during PTCA procedures such as the TandemHeart and the investigational Impella device. Furthermore, the evolution of drug-eluting stents has dramatically reduced restenosis rates. The evolution of successful revascularization techniques may be complicated by the presence of microvascular dysfunction and the search continues for minimally invasive approaches that provide long-term benefits in challenging patients such as the diabetic.

The future may hold more advanced technologies that utilize gene therapy as an inhibitor of restenosis. Studies have documented that local gene

transfer of tissue factor pathway inhibitor regulated intimal hyperplasia in atherosclerotic arteries [23]. Transfer of fortilin, an anti-apoptotic protein, results in suppression of vascular smooth muscle cell proliferation and migration [24]. Moreover, gene transduction has been shown to result in increased blood flow and decreased restenosis after injury in diseased vessels [25]. This concept of local gene transduction will play a major role in the future of revascularization procedures.

Restore Function to Infarcted Myocardium via Replacement of Non-functional Myocardium or the Entire Heart

Targeting the energy metabolism of the human heart is another modality for treatment of ischemic disease that will become an important treatment option. The human heart requires the highest oxygen uptake in the body ($\sim$0.1 mL O_2/g/min at rest) and consumes about 6 kg of adenosine triphosphate (ATP)/day. The ATP content of the cardiac myocyte is $<$ 1 gram. Thus, these cells must produce large amounts of ATP to maintain normal energetics. To facilitate this, cardiac myocytes have the highest mitochondrial density in the body and can utilize multiple substrates to generate energy including fatty acids, ketones, and carbohydrates. There is an energy reserve compound known as phosphocreatine (PCr) that rapidly regenerates ATP when an abrupt demand is placed on the heart. PCr has been found to decrease in heart failure, a catabolic process, which results in a further ATP depleted environment leading to a resultant depletion of ATP in end-stage heart failure [26, 27]. Thus, impaired energy use in the heart plays a significant role in the progression of heart failure [28] and targeting the mitochondria and energetics of myocytes will be a consideration in the future management of heart failure.

Substrates change in the setting of heart failure as the heart utilizes less fatty acid metabolism and relies more on carbohydrates [29]. Perhaps by shifting cell use back to fatty acids or optimizing the use of carbohydrates, cardiac function can be improved. The attempt to up-regulate fatty acid metabolism in animal models may have detrimental effects perhaps secondary to increased potential for lipotoxicity [30, 31]. Another possible future application may be partially inhibiting fatty acid oxidation, which may lead to an increased use of glucose [32, 33]. This may be useful, as rescue of cells deficient in enzymes necessary for fatty acid metabolism with increased levels of the glucose transporter GLUT1 improved left ventricular function in animal models of dilated cardiomyopathy [34]. There are medicines that are currently in use for the treatment of diabetes that improve insulin sensitivity such as metformin. Although the use of these medicines in heart failure has been considered potentially harmful [35], observational data has documented an improvement in outcomes in older patients with heart failure and diabetes [36]. A large scale clinical trial is warranted to evaluate the impacts that alterations in the energetics of the failing myocardium may have.

The concept of cell-based cardiac repair has gained a large amount of focus over the past decade and is discussed in previous chapters. This modality will only become more widely used in the future. There have been several studies utilizing skeletal muscle in ischemic cardiomyopathy [37–39]. No conclusions can be made but there are some indications of improvement in function but arrhythmias have been a concern.

The use of bone marrow has also been explored in chronic ischemic disease [40–42]. Results are striking but with the small sample sizes of the studies, the results are difficult to interpret. There is a difficulty in choosing the correct cell line. An ideal cell population would (1) be readily and widely available, (2) have the ability to generate new cardiac myocytes, (3) be able to directly or indirectly generate new coronary vasculature, (4) result in a small amount of scar between the host myocardium and the transplanted cells, (5) proliferate to fill in areas of dysfunctional myocardium, and (6) be accepted by the host immune system [43]. This approach will also require a novel design for cell delivery that is innovative. Such a system would result in generation of funds to propel the research of cell-based cardiac repair to a higher level. With the intense use of resources in this area, perhaps the problem of "ideal lineages" will be surmountable.

Generation of "cellular scaffolding" is a concept with appeal. By removing dysfunctional cardiac myocytes, a skeleton remains which could serve as a lattice that could be repopulated with healthy, functional cells (Fig. 8.3). One application of this technology is the development of a human fibroblast-based, tissue-engineered, epicardial patch. When applied to an ischemic area of the heart, the living tissue provides cytokines and growth factors needed to induce angiogenesis (blood vessel formation) and tissue repair. This is an active, exciting area of research that could lend valuable information in the generation of an entire heart that could be the "perfect match" for transplantation.

Mechanically Supporting the Failing or Ischemic Heart Without Surgery

Current long-term mechanical support devices such as left ventricular assist devices (LVADs) require use of the heart lung machine and extensive surgery. The

A

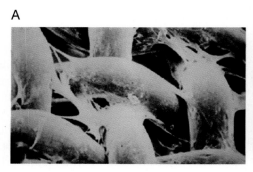

B

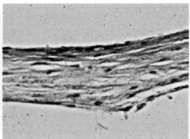

Fig. 8.3 (A) Human fibroblast stretching across the three-dimensional scaffold composed of Vicryl suture material, a biodegradable sugar polymer. (B) Histological cross-section of anginera (a human fibroblast-based, tissue-engineered, epicardial patch) showing fibroblast cells and matrix they have made. The cells are alive and secrete growth factors

modern patient with chronic heart failure, who represents the largest population in need of such devices, is often plagued with comorbid illnesses, chronic cachexia, and debilitation and therefore may not tolerate extensive surgery. The future will see mechanical support devices that will be implantable without use of the heart lung machine and in fact may be implantable without general anesthesia in a catheterization laboratory setting. Such devices will utilize small axial or centrifugal pumps, which will only partially unload the ventricle, thus allowing for myocardial recovery and improvement of ischemia.

One such design is Exalaras device from Orqis medical, which extracts blood from the distal aorta and pumps into the proximal descending aorta, thus accelerating blood flow in the descending aorta and providing greater splanchnic and renal perfusion while gently unloading the left ventricle. This device is in the preclinical phase and is slated for human implant in 2008. Another preclinical device made by CircuLite Corporation draws blood from the left atrium through an intravascularly placed cannula to a subclavian site that houses the pump, which then pumps blood into an arterial cannula in the subclavian artery. The device unloads the ventricle while contributing to total forward cardiac output. A third concept only device is being developed at the Texas Heart Institute and involves the use of a very small micro axial flow pump, which is implanted in the lumen of the descending or ascending aorta and anchored via a strut system. This device could be catheter delivered and may unload the ventricle by decreasing afterload and improving distal organ perfusion. The drive line supplying electrical power to this device would exit the arterial system at the site of implant and attach to a subcutaneously implanted rechargeable battery or transcutaneous energy transmission system. These concepts are in the very early stages of development but offer hope in the future for servicing the real patient with chronic heart failure and chronic coronary disease that we face in amazingly high numbers today.

Advances in microminiaturization of pumps, battery technology, and transcutaneous energy transmission may make these concepts a reality in the near future. It is now possible to make a pump that is as small as a pencil eraser deliver 5 l/min of blood flow and both axial and centrifugal pumps are being developed with magnetically levitated rotors, which eliminate problems with bearing wear and longevity of use. Battery design has improved in both efficiency and size, and the old technology of transcutaneous energy transmission, in which an external induction coil recharges an internal battery without touching it or breaking the skin, has already seen clinical use in surgically implanted devices. Thus, it is likely that the left ventricular mechanical unloading devices of the future will be implantable via a procedure similar in scope to a current defibrillator implant.

Devices such as this could potentially be applied to a much larger population of patients than the surgical LVADs currently in use because the morbidity and mortality associated with the minimally invasive implant technique may be greatly reduced. As a result, such devices could be used as a bridge to recovery of function in ischemic or post myocardial infarction or acute myocarditis. In addition, the larger population of patients with chronic heart failure may benefit from the use of these devices earlier in the course of disease to prevent progression to end stage heart failure. Finally, such devices could be used as an adjunct to support function while other procedures are performed such as high risk revascularization or stem cell implant. With the advent of defibrillators that monitor hemodynamic parameters, feedback data to alter pump outputs according to physiologic need may be achievable. There is no question that in the future the implantation methods of mechanical support devices will evolve, as so many other cardiovascular procedures have, to less invasive techniques.

Better Utilize Existing Technologies to Slow or Prevent the Progression of the Disease

Part of the futuristic approach to treating advanced ischemic heart disease will encompass a better understanding of and better utilization of existing technologies that previously were not considered to be beneficial. We can and should explore simple technologies and techniques used for other disease states to augment the treatment of this disease. Much effort has been placed in the research of coronary biology and ischemic heart disease. However, over the past few decades, the appreciation for the complex interplay between the heart and other organ systems has grown. The neurochemical and hemodynamic stress placed on the heart by extra-cardiac processes has been a focus of treatment with secondary results on cardiac causes of morbidity and mortality.

Medical therapy continues to be an important tool in the management of ischemic heart failure. However, considerations to the type of therapy used remain unusually broad and guideline based. Patients with heart failure, regardless of etiology, are currently managed along a typical, predictable algorithm that is tailored to patients based on symptoms, clinical findings, and side-effect profiles. However, one must consider the possibility that all patients may not respond similarly to a given regimen of oral or intravenous therapies. It is well documented in large scale clinical trials that non-responders exist. This has been reported extensively on a cellular level with non-responders to aspirin therapy.

It must be remembered that results of clinical trials, regardless of design or outcome, do not focus on the response to therapy per individual. Instead, the clinical trial results reflect a very heterogenous mix of patients that have the potential for various responses based on genotypic and phenotypic factors. The inherent problem is that there are no accepted and validated methods for assessing the potential differences in response to standard approaches to the use of ACE inhibition, beta blockade, aldosterone antagonism, or other medical strategies. Perhaps even the sequential approach that we currently follow may be more effective if delivered in a different order [44]. The future management ischemic heart failure may include more individually tailored therapies that are based on analysis of temporal and physiologic changes that are a part of the dynamic nature of the disease.

Vast amounts of resources and time are being devoted to proteomics. Proteomics, a term referring to the entire group of *pro*teins associated with a given gen*ome*, may offer insight into this complicated problem. Use of proteomics is widely used in current-day cardiology. Cardiac-specific troponins, structural proteins found uniquely in the cardiomyocyte, are used in the diagnosis of myocardial

injury. B-type natriuretic peptide (BNP), a protein synthesized in the heart in response to left ventricular wall tension, is used in the diagnosis and management of various cardiac and non-cardiac processes such as heart failure, acute coronary syndromes, and pulmonary embolism. C-reactive protein (CRP), a marker of inflammation made in the liver, is being used as an indicator of risk for atherosclerosis, which is, at least in part, an inflammatory process. This, however, only begins to touch on the potential for use of such proteins. Future work involving proteomics could greatly enhance the identification and utilization of these markers. Many of the markers available now and potentially in the future are very low abundance proteins in the blood. For example, tumor necrosis factor alpha (TNFα) is a predictor of outcomes in the setting of heart failure and is the target for potential antagonism. However, the circulating levels of TNFα are in the femtomolar range (10^{-15}).

The use of markers such as those listed is already widely used. A large reason for this use is the ease and availability of blood samples. Blood testing is also relatively inexpensive and testing can be performed in hospitals globally. Furthermore, serologic testing is a logical focus as most all cells use the blood to communicate with each other offering a partial understanding of the complex interrelationships between organ systems such as the endocrine and renal effects on the heart. The use of artificial intelligence paradigms may allow this to be possible on a larger scale. This has already been shown to be effective in the detection of ovarian cancer.

Clinical outcomes could be favorably altered by using this technology to evaluate *individual* patients at a specific point in their course to assess complex protein interactions to design specific therapy *unique to each patient*. By doing so, time and resources could be saved and potential adverse effects of unnecessary and potentially harmful therapy could be avoided. The other exciting possibility of this approach is that management could be altered more rapidly and efficaciously as these proteomic profiles change over time. It must be remembered that the genome is a relatively stable entity as is the proteins derived from the transcription of DNA to mRNA and translation into proteins. However, the resultant milieu of proteins and their interplay at the cellular level is a constantly changing dynamic, thus representing a "snap-shot" of a cell or group of cells at a single point in time.

There are obvious problems associated with the clinical application of proteomics that must be answered. First, proteins must be identified and described with respect to function and physiologic impact. Second, consensus is necessary regarding the testing and reporting of the proteins. Third, the implementation of the technology would require wide-spread access with an economically feasible method of delivery. Last, the methods would need to be reproducible and valid. The potential for the use of such technology is very likely in the next few decades and will have significant impact on the lives of heart failure patients.

More effective screening and treatment of comorbidities commonly seen in heart failure may contribute significant gains. Anemia is a common finding in heart failure, typically normochromic and normocytic. It is felt to be an anemia of chronic disease but the exact mechanism remains unclear but may be related to increases in N-acetyl-seryl-aspartyl-lysyl-proline (Ac-SDKP), an inhibitor of hematopoeisis. (van de meer circ 2005) The definition of anemia varies, but it has been reported that hemoglobin levels between 10–12 g/dL cause an increase in exercise cardiac output. This results in left ventricular workload and cardiomyocyte oxygen consumption, which leads to accelerated loss of cardiac muscle [45]. Anemia has been widely recognized in heart failure patients with a varying prevalence of 22–39% [46, 47].

The mechanism of anemia in heart failure is multifactorial. Cytokines have been implicated in the process, specifically TNFα. TNF-a has been shown to blunt the production and proliferation of erythroid progenitors [48]. The drug therapies used for heart failure also may contribute to anemia. ACE inhibitors and ARBs have been shown to result in a decrease in angioitensin-II receptor mediated activity [49, 50]. This relationship is further augmented by evidence of communication by the same second messenger system, Jak STAT [51, 52].

The impact of anemia on outcomes in heart failure is well documented. Horwich et al. documented a 16% increased risk of death with each 1 g/dL decrease in hemoglobin [53]. Secondary to these findings, erythropoietin (EPO) has been used in

randomized opne-label studies. Silverberg and colleagues have reported that correction of hemoglobin from 10 mg/dL to 12 mg/dL with subcutaneous EPO and intravenous iron resulted in a significant improvement in functional class and ejection fraction with a reduction in need for diuretic therapy [54].

The evaluation and treatment of anemia in heart failure is still in the early stages. The use of EPO in patients with NYHA Class III–IV heart failure was well tolerated in a study by Mancini et al., with an increase in hemoglobin and exercise capacity [55]. The postulated mechanism of improvement in VO2 is increased oxygen delivery secondary to increased hemoglobin concentrations. Although the long term outcomes of treatment with iron supplementation and EPO are still not known, current data suggest that treatment of anemia may improve symptoms and systolic function. Further investigation is needed as anemia has been clearly defined as a marker for increased mortality in these patients.

Obesity continues to be a major health crisis in developed nations with alarming trends toward increasing obesity in the United States. Obesity has been shown to be a risk factor for left ventricular remodeling as well as left ventricular hypertrophy and dilatation, which are well recognized predictors of heart failure [56–59]. Obesity is an important risk factor for developing heart failure with approximately 11% of cases of heart failure among men and 14% among women in the community are attributable to obesity alone [60]. Moreover, avoidance of obesity and overweight in adult life in both men with and without CHD may reduce their later risk of total and coronary heart disease mortality [61]. More aggressive recognition, counseling, and treatment by primary and specialty health-care providers of obesity may ameliorate this concerning trend.

Obstructive sleep apnea (OSA), which is typically characterized by intermittent hypoxia/reoxygenation (IHR), is a common finding in patients with heart failure and is an independent risk factor for cardiovascular disease [62–64]. OSA has been shown to result in activation of selective markers of inflammation, which could be the basis of the molecular mechanism of the cardiovascular disease seen in these patients [65]. The OSA syndrome has been shown to significantly increase the risk of stroke or death from any cause independent of other risk factors such as hypertension [66]. Thus, the effective treatment of OSA may ultimately have far-reaching impacts on outcomes in patients with heart failure.

A study from the CANPAP investigators evaluated the hypothesis that continuous airway pressure (CPAP) would improve survival rates in patients with the comorbid diagnoses of heart failure and sleep apnea [67]. Their study revealed an improvement in nocturnal oxygenation, increased LV ejection fractions, and increased distance walked in 6 min. However, there was no change in survival at 18 months. The study did show a divergence in the control versus CPAP groups at 60 months and lacked power to demonstrate with certainty that CPAP is ineffective in this population. Perhaps this may portend a significant benefit over time. Other studies have also documented improvement in LV ejection fraction as well as reducing levels of atrial natriuretic peptide (ANP) and norepinephrine and improving assessed patient quality of life [68–70]. These favorable changes in neurohormonal profiles may have significant impacts on these patients. Future studies with longer follow-up and broader assessment of quality of life are warranted.

Detect and Monitor Established Heart Failure or Ischemia

In the near future it will be possible to monitor the status of heart failure using sensors incorporated in the newest generations of defibrillators. Major manufacturers of these devices have put in them the ability to monitor such parameters as heart rate variability, pressure in the right ventricle and force of contraction of the heart as well as many other parameters that are of as yet uncertain significance. As experience with using these data increases the ability to ascertain their utility in the management of patients will increase.

The data recorded by these novel defibrillators can be downloaded in the office of the general and heart failure cardiologist with a simple device that will provide a printout of a "heart failure profile," which can be used in the assessment of the patient at that clinic visit. This has been demonstrated by the

COMPASS investigators. In COMPASS, an implantable device that continuously monitors intra-cardiac pressures was shown to be safe and to improve care in patients with chronic heart failure [71]. Some simple measured parameters such as activity of the patient and heart rate and respiratory rate can be plotted over time to determine the patient's level of activity and provide insight into their functional status.

The challenge is to be able to use the data from these defibrillators to prevent admissions to the hospital by detecting decompensation early. In addition, it is hoped that they will aid in following the progression of the disease and thus help determine need for advanced therapy options such as transplant or mechanical support. Data has also been recorded evaluating impedance as a marker of lung wetness [72]. This information may give sufficient "warning" to clinicians to avert hospital admissions by altering management strategies. Challenges exist in how to best use and communicate the data outside of the routine clinic visit to prevent additional burdens to the already busy job of the practicing clinician.

Conclusion

Broad areas of research that we may see in the not too distant future include gene therapy and nanotechnology. Gene therapy is a natural approach to the problem of advanced ischemic heart disease. Genetic manipulations have the potential to improve myocardial function, promote neoangiogenesis, and protect the heart from ischemic injury. Genes can be transferred to the heart by multilple mechanisms including intracoronary injection to affect the coronary vascular endothelium, viral vectors that migrate to the myocardium and deliver genes of interest, and direct delivery of genes during coronary angioplasty and stent placement.

Much work has been done in the area of vascular growth factors to create collateral circulation, but so far clinical efforts have fallen short of predictions. The new field of cell transplantation may provide the necessary milieu and may be more effective at inducing neovascularization in ischemic myocardium. Fibroblast growth factor in intracoronary injections is being studied for its ability to improve myocardial ischemia in patients with distal disease, which is difficult to revascularize by standard means. As diabetic vascular disease increases in incidence this has an exciting potential.

A powerful new line of research involves using viral vectors such as adenovirus to infect the myocardium in an effort to improve function. An intravascular injection using homing mechanisms and direct epicardial injection are being studied. Many molecular derangements occur in the failing myocardium that may be potentially reversed with gene introduction. Gene introduction via coronary catheters is being studied for re-stenosis and particularly for prevention or treatment of vein graft disease. Beta receptor modulation may be another target for gene therapy and early studies designed at this approach are under way. Finally, cardiomyopathy due to inborn errors of metabolism may also be a target. As gene regulation is involved, either directly or indirectly, in initiation or progression of cardiac disease, this will remain a potential therapeutic target for the future.

The ability to create smaller and smaller molecules and devices (nanotechnology) opens new possibilities for many fields of medicine. For example, scientists have created in the laboratory an organic molecule that when heated, linked compounds move in alternation so that it can move in a straight line across a smooth surface. In a test, such a molecule took 10,000 "steps" [73]. If we can make a molecule that can walk, then it should be possible to synthetically recreate the sarcomere to some extent and possibly build "synthetic muscle."

We now have entirely new ways of thinking about advanced ischemic heart disease and heart failure and this has opened up a bright future for new treatments. For example, if we can use new measures to decrease the workload of the heart, then it is clear that in many patients that heart failure progression and possibly reversal may occur. This is a major breakthrough in the thinking of the pathophysiology of heart failure. It has also become clear recently that the heart has significant potential to adapt to the ischemic condition and this has created new targets for therapy. Finally, revascularization technologies and techniques continue to evolve leaving only very few patients without a revascularization option.

Consider scenarios such as these: a patient presents with intractable angina after prior bypass surgery and has no revascularization option. At the time of his bypass stem cells were stored for future use and are implanted non-surgically along with factors to promote neovascularization in conduits created in the ischemic zone. In a second case a patient presents with heart failure and extensive non-viability and a temporary percutaneous assist pump is implanted while myocardial tissue is engineered from harvested stem cells for later grafting to the non-viable sites. These are examples of the hope we have of treating patients so that no one will have to die while waiting for a transplant or suffer the impaired quality of life associated with angina and heart failure. In the coming years we will be able to offer hope where none existed before.

When we think about the future of the treatment of complex cardiovascular disease, there are two things to consider: first, what we can do and second, what we should do. Our abilities to design new therapies with advances in engineering, pharmacology, and genetics is growing at a tremendous rate, perhaps faster than we have the ability to apply those therapies to practice. Thus, we must focus on making highly advanced technology practical and affordable to the health care system. This means simplification, miniaturization, and ease of deployment. Successful new therapies should be easy to employ using standard technologies, easy to monitor, and applicable in existing medical care facilities. Non-surgical solutions are needed due to the tremendous burden of surgery on the already chronically ill patient and the long recovery times necessary. Cell and gene therapies should be easily produced and stored and medicines should be inexpensive and without complex monitoring and dosing. As new technologies come to patient use, the three major contributors to the care of the patient—the caregiver, the "payor," and the federal regulatory system—should work in concert in a collaborative manner to achieve these goals. Finally, in using new therapies, it is important to consider the effects of the therapy on mortality, progression of the disease, on quality of life, and cost. We have a responsibility to never forget the end goal to improve the longevity and quality of life of the patient living with advanced heart disease and to do it in a way that leave no one in need.

The final thought in editing this textbook is to never forget the most important intervention we can make as caregivers and that is prevention. Greater appreciation must be given to those patients that are increased risk of developing ischemic cardiac disease and resultant heart failure [1]. Education of health-care professionals and patients alike is critical to utilizing this tool to the greatest potential. The most powerful thing we can do to impact the lives of people and the viability of the health care system is to prevent disease and this is what we must have foremost on our mind in treating people with heart disease.

References

1. Hunt SA, Abraham WT, Chin MH, et al. ACC/AHA 2005 Guideline Update for the Diagnosis and Management of Chronic Heart Failure in the Adult-Summary Article A Report of the American College of Cardiology/American Heart Association Task Force on Practice Guidelines (Writing Committee to Update the 2001 Guidelines for the Evaluation and Management of Heart Failure). *J Am Coll Cardiol*. Sep 20 2005;46(6):1116–1143.
2. Levy D, Kenchaiah S, Larson MG, et al. Long-term trends in the incidence of and survival with heart failure. *N Engl J Med*. Oct 31 2002;347(18):1397–1402.
3. Schlegel TT, Kulecz WB, DePalma JL, et al. Real-time 12-lead high-frequency QRS electrocardiography for enhanced detection of myocardial ischemia and coronary artery disease. *Mayo Clin Proc*. Mar 2004;79(3):339–350.
4. Vrtovec B, Starc V, Starc R. Beat-to-beat QT interval variability in coronary patients. *J Electrocardiol*. Apr 2000;33(2):119–125.
5. Topol EJ. Simon Dack Lecture. The genomic basis of myocardial infarction. *J Am Coll Cardiol*. Oct 18 2005;46(8):1456–1465.
6. Pajukanta P, Cargill M, Viitanen L, et al. Two loci on chromosomes 2 and X for premature coronary heart disease identified in early- and late-settlement populations of Finland. *Am J Hum Genet*. Dec 2000;67(6):1481–1493.
7. Francke S, Manraj M, Lacquemant C, et al. A genome-wide scan for coronary heart disease suggests in Indo-Mauritians a susceptibility locus on chromosome 16p13 and replicates linkage with the metabolic syndrome on 3q27. *Hum Mol Genet*. Nov 15 2001;10(24):2751–2765.
8. Broeckel U, Hengstenberg C, Mayer B, et al. A comprehensive linkage analysis for myocardial infarction and its related risk factors. *Nat Genet*. Feb 2002;30(2):210–214.
9. Harrap SB, Zammit KS, Wong ZY, et al. Genome-wide linkage analysis of the acute coronary syndrome suggests a locus on chromosome 2. *Arterioscler Thromb Vasc Biol*. May 1 2002;22(5):874–878.
10. Hauser ER, Crossman DC, Granger CB, et al. A genomewide scan for early-onset coronary artery disease in 438 families: the GENECARD Study. *Am J Hum Genet*. Sep 2004;75(3):436–447.
11. Wang Q, Rao S, Shen GQ, et al. Premature myocardial infarction novel susceptibility locus on chromosome 1P34–36 identified by genomewide linkage analysis. *Am J Hum Genet*. Feb 2004;74(2):262–271.
12. Helgadottir A, Manolescu A, Thorleifsson G, et al. The gene encoding 5-lipoxygenase activating protein confers risk of myocardial infarction and stroke. *Nat Genet*. Mar 2004;36(3):233–239.
13. Wang L, Fan C, Topol SE, et al. Mutation of MEF2A in an inherited disorder with features of coronary artery disease. *Science*. Nov 28 2003;302(5650):1578–1581.
14. Towbin JA. The role of cytoskeletal proteins in cardiomyopathies. *Curr Opin Cell Biol*. Feb 1998;10(1):131–139.
15. Hoffman EP, Brown RH, Jr., Kunkel LM. Dystrophin: the protein product of the Duchenne muscular dystrophy locus. *Cell*. Dec 24 1987;51(6):919–928.
16. Vatta M, Stetson SJ, Jimenez S, et al. Molecular normalization of dystrophin in the failing left and right ventricle of patients treated with either pulsatile or continuous flow-type ventricular assist devices. *J Am Coll Cardiol*. Mar 3 2004;43(5):811–817.
17. Vatta M, Stetson SJ, Perez-Verdia A, et al. Molecular remodelling of dystrophin in patients with end-stage cardiomyopathies and reversal in patients on assistance-device therapy. *Lancet*. Mar 16 2002;359(9310):936–941.
18. Badorff C, Lee GH, Lamphear BJ, et al. Enteroviral protease 2A cleaves dystrophin: evidence of cytoskeletal disruption in an acquired cardiomyopathy. *Nat Med*. Mar 1999;5(3):320–326.
19. Jefferies JL, Eidem BW, Belmont JW, et al. Genetic predictors and remodeling of dilated cardiomyopathy in muscular dystrophy. *Circulation*. Nov 1 2005;112(18):2799–2804.
20. Monraats PS, Pires NM, Agema WR, et al. Genetic inflammatory factors predict restenosis after percutaneous coronary interventions. *Circulation*. Oct 18 2005;112(16):2417–2425.
21. Levy D, Larson MG, Vasan RS, et al. The progression from hypertension to congestive heart failure. *JAMA*. May 22–29 1996;275(20):1557–1562.
22. Adamson PB, Abraham WT, Love C, et al. The evolving challenge of chronic heart failure management: a call for a new curriculum for training heart failure specialists. *J Am Coll Cardiol*. Oct 6 2004;44(7):1354–1357.
23. Zoldhelyi P, Chen ZQ, Shelat HS, et al. Local gene transfer of tissue factor pathway inhibitor regulates intimal hyperplasia in atherosclerotic arteries. *Proc Natl Acad Sci U S A*. Mar 27 2001;98(7):4078–4083.
24. Tulis DA, Mnjoyan ZH, Schiesser RL, et al. Adenoviral gene transfer of fortilin attenuates neointima formation through suppression of vascular smooth muscle cell proliferation and migration. *Circulation*. Jan 7 2003;107(1):98–105.

25. Liu Q, Chen ZQ, Bobustuc GC, et al. Local gene trans-
    duction of cyclooxygenase-1 increases blood flow in
    injured atherosclerotic rabbit arteries. *Circulation*. Apr
    12 2005;111(14):1833–1840.
26. Tian R, Nascimben L, Kaddurah-Daouk R, et al.
    Depletion of energy reserve via the creatine kinase reac-
    tion during the evolution of heart failure in cardiomyo-
    pathic hamsters. *J Mol Cell Cardiol*. Apr 1996;28(4):
    755–765.
27. Neubauer S, Horn M, Cramer M, et al. Myocardial
    phosphocreatine-to-ATP ratio is a predictor of mortality
    in patients with dilated cardiomyopathy. *Circulation*.
    Oct 7 1997;96(7):2190–2196.
28. Taegtmeyer H, Wilson CR, Razeghi P, et al. Metabolic
    energetics and genetics in the heart. *Ann N Y Acad Sci*.
    Jun 2005;1047:208–218.
29. Sambandam N, Lopaschuk GD, Brownsey RW, et al.
    Energy metabolism in the hypertrophied heart. *Heart
    Fail Rev*. Apr 2002;7(2):161–173.
30. Dewald O, Sharma S, Adrogue J, et al. Downregulation
    of peroxisome proliferator-activated receptor-alpha
    gene expression in a mouse model of ischemic
    cardiomyopathy is dependent on reactive oxygen
    species and prevents lipotoxicity. *Circulation*. Jul 19
    2005;112(3):407–415.
31. Young ME, Laws FA, Goodwin GW, et al. Reactivation
    of peroxisome proliferator-activated receptor alpha
    is associated with contractile dysfunction in hyper-
    trophied rat heart. *J Biol Chem*. Nov 30 2001;
    276(48):44390–44395.
32. Kantor PF, Lucien A, Kozak R, et al. The antianginal
    drug trimetazidine shifts cardiac energy metabolism
    from fatty acid oxidation to glucose oxidation by inhibit-
    ing mitochondrial long-chain 3-ketoacyl coenzyme A
    thiolase. *Circ Res*. Mar 17 2000;86(5):580–588.
33. Lopaschuk GD. Optimizing cardiac energy metabolism:
    how can fatty acid and carbohydrate metabolism be
    manipulated? *Coron Artery Dis*. Feb 2001;12 Suppl
    1:S8–11.
34. Nikolaidis LA, Elahi D, Hentosz T, et al. Recombinant
    glucagon-like peptide-1 increases myocardial glucose
    uptake and improves left ventricular performance in
    conscious dogs with pacing-induced dilated cardiomyo-
    pathy. *Circulation*. Aug 24 2004;110(8):955–961.
35. Nesto RW, Bell D, Bonow RO, et al. Thiazolidinedione
    use, fluid retention, and congestive heart failure: a con-
    sensus statement from the American Heart Association
    and American Diabetes Association. October 7, 2003.
    Circulation. Dec 9 2003;108(23):2941–2948.
36. Masoudi FA, Inzucchi SE, Wang Y, et al. Thiazolidine-
    diones, metformin, and outcomes in older patients with
    diabetes and heart failure: an observational study. *Cir-
    culation*. Feb 8 2005;111(5):583–590.
37. Menasche P, Hagege AA, Vilquin JT, et al. Autologous
    skeletal myoblast transplantation for severe postinfarc-
    tion left ventricular dysfunction. *J Am Coll Cardiol*. Apr
    2 2003;41(7):1078–1083.
38. Herreros J, Prosper F, Perez A, et al. Autologous intra-
    myocardial injection of cultured skeletal muscle-derived
    stem cells in patients with non-acute myocardial infarc-
    tion. *Eur Heart J*. Nov 2003;24(22):2012–2020.

39. Siminiak T, Kalawski R, Fiszer D, et al. Autologous
    skeletal myoblast transplantation for the treatment of
    postinfarction myocardial injury: phase I clinical study
    with 12 months of follow-up. *Am Heart J*. Sep
    2004;148(3):531–537.
40. Tse HF, Kwong YL, Chan JK, et al. Angiogenesis in
    ischaemic myocardium by intramyocardial autologous
    bone marrow mononuclear cell implantation. *Lancet*.
    Jan 4 2003;361(9351):47–49.
41. Perin EC, Dohmann HF, Borojevic R, et al. Transendo-
    cardial, autologous bone marrow cell transplantation for
    severe, chronic ischemic heart failure. *Circulation*. May
    13 2003;107(18):2294–2302.
42. Fuchs S, Satler LF, Kornowski R, et al. Catheter-based
    autologous bone marrow myocardial injection in no-
    option patients with advanced coronary artery disease:
    a feasibility study. *J Am Coll Cardiol*. May 21
    2003;41(10):1721–1724.
43. Murry CE, Field LJ, Menasche P. Cell-based cardiac
    repair: reflections at the 10-year point. *Circulation*. Nov
    15 2005;112(20):3174–3183.
44. Willenheimer R, van Veldhuisen DJ, Silke B, et al.
    Effect on survival and hospitalization of initiating treat-
    ment for chronic heart failure with bisoprolol followed
    by enalapril, as compared with the opposite sequence:
    results of the randomized Cardiac Insufficiency Biso-
    prolol Study (CIBIS) III. *Circulation*. Oct 18
    2005;112(16):2426–2435.
45. Metivier F, Marchais SJ, Guerin AP, et al. Pathophysiol-
    ogy of anaemia: focus on the heart and blood vessels.
    Nephrol Dial Transplant. 2000;15 Suppl 3:14–18.
46. Al-Ahmad A, Rand WM, Manjunath G, et al. Reduced
    kidney function and anemia as risk factors for mortality
    in patients with left ventricular dysfunction. *J Am Coll
    Cardiol*. Oct 2001;38(4):955–962.
47. Kalra PR, Bolger AP, Francis DP, et al. Effect of anemia
    on exercise tolerance in chronic heart failure in men. *Am
    J Cardiol*. Apr 1 2003;91(7):888–891.
48. Iversen PO, Woldbaek PR, Tonnessen T, et al.
    Decreased hematopoiesis in bone marrow of mice with
    congestive heart failure. *Am J Physiol Regul Integr Comp
    Physiol*. Jan 2002;282(1):R166–172.
49. Mrug M, Stopka T, Julian BA, et al. Angiotensin II
    stimulates proliferation of normal early erythroid pro-
    genitors. *J Clin Invest*. Nov 1 1997;100(9):2310–2314.
50. Rodgers KE, Xiong S, Steer R, et al. Effect of angioten-
    sin II on hematopoietic progenitor cell proliferation.
    Stem Cells. 2000;18(4):287–294.
51. Cole J, Ertoy D, Lin H, et al. Lack of angiotensin II-
    facilitated erythropoiesis causes anemia in angiotensin-
    converting enzyme-deficient mice. *J Clin Invest*. Dec
    2000;106(11):1391–1398.
52. Mrug M, Julian BA, Prchal JT. Angiotensin II receptor
    type 1 expression in erythroid progenitors: Implications
    for the pathogenesis of postrenal transplant erythrocy-
    tosis. *Semin Nephrol*. Mar 2004;24(2):120–130.
53. Horwich TB, Fonarow GC, Hamilton MA, et al. Ane-
    mia is associated with worse symptoms, greater impair-
    ment in functional capacity and a significant increase in
    mortality in patients with advanced heart failure. *J Am
    Coll Cardiol*. Jun 5 2002;39(11):1780–1786.

54. Silverberg DS, Wexler D, Blum M, et al. The use of subcutaneous erythropoietin and intravenous iron for the treatment of the anemia of severe, resistant congestive heart failure improves cardiac and renal function and functional cardiac class, and markedly reduces hospitalizations. *J Am Coll Cardiol.* Jun 2000;35(7):1737–1744.

55. Mancini DM, Katz SD, Lang CC, et al. Effect of erythropoietin on exercise capacity in patients with moderate to severe chronic heart failure. *Circulation.* Jan 21 2003;107(2): 294–299.

56. Messerli FH, Sundgaard-Riise K, Reisin ED, et al. Dimorphic cardiac adaptation to obesity and arterial hypertension. *Ann Intern Med.* Dec 1983;99(6):757–761.

57. Hammond IW, Devereux RB, Alderman MH, et al. Relation of blood pressure and body build to left ventricular mass in normotensive and hypertensive employed adults. *J Am Coll Cardiol.* Oct 1988;12(4):996–1004.

58. Lauer MS, Anderson KM, Kannel WB, et al. The impact of obesity on left ventricular mass and geometry. The Framingham Heart Study. *JAMA.* Jul 10 1991;266(2):231–236.

59. Alpert MA, Lambert CR, Terry BE, et al. Influence of left ventricular mass on left ventricular diastolic filling in normotensive morbid obesity. *Am Heart J.* Nov 1995;130(5):1068–1073.

60. Kenchaiah S, Evans JC, Levy D, et al. Obesity and the risk of heart failure. *N Engl J Med.* Aug 1 2002;347(5):305–313.

61. Batty GD, Shipley M, Jarrett J, et al. Obesity and overweight in relation to disease-specific mortality in men with and without existing coronary heart disease in London: The original Whitehall study. *Heart.* Nov 3 2005.

62. Bradley TD, Floras JS. Sleep apnea and heart failure: Part II: central sleep apnea. *Circulation.* Apr 8 2003;107(13):1822–1826.

63. Sin DD, Fitzgerald F, Parker JD, et al. Risk factors for central and obstructive sleep apnea in 450 men and women with congestive heart failure. *Am J Respir Crit Care Med.* Oct 1999;160(4):1101–1106.

64. Lanfranchi PA, Braghiroli A, Bosimini E, et al. Prognostic value of nocturnal Cheyne-Stokes respiration in chronic heart failure. *Circulation.* Mar 23 1999;99(11):1435–1440.

65. Ryan S, Taylor CT, McNicholas WT. Selective activation of inflammatory pathways by intermittent hypoxia in obstructive sleep apnea syndrome. *Circulation.* Oct 25 2005;112(17):2660–2667.

66. Yaggi HK, Concato J, Kernan WN, et al. Obstructive sleep apnea as a risk factor for stroke and death. *N Engl J Med.* Nov 10 2005;353(19):2034–2041.

67. Bradley TD, Logan AG, Kimoff RJ, et al. Continuous positive airway pressure for central sleep apnea and heart failure. *N Engl J Med.* Nov 10 2005;353(19):2025–2033.

68. Naughton MT, Liu PP, Bernard DC, et al. Treatment of congestive heart failure and Cheyne-Stokes respiration during sleep by continuous positive airway pressure. *Am J Respir Crit Care Med.* Jan 1995;151(1):92–97.

69. Tkacova R, Liu PP, Naughton MT, et al. Effect of continuous positive airway pressure on mitral regurgitant fraction and atrial natriuretic peptide in patients with heart failure. *J Am Coll Cardiol.* Sep 1997;30(3):739–745.

70. Naughton MT, Benard DC, Liu PP, et al. Effects of nasal CPAP on sympathetic activity in patients with heart failure and central sleep apnea. *Am J Respir Crit Care Med.* Aug 1995;152(2):473–479.

71. Cleland JG, Coletta AP, Freemantle N, et al. Clinical trials update from the American College of Cardiology meeting: CARE-HF and the remission of heart failure, Women's Health Study, TNT, COMPASS-HF, VERITAS, CANPAP, PEECH and PREMIER. *Eur J Heart Fail.* Aug 2005;7(5):931–936.

72. Yu CM, Wang L, Chau E, et al. Intrathoracic impedance monitoring in patients with heart failure: correlation with fluid status and feasibility of early warning preceding hospitalization. *Circulation.* Aug 9 2005;112(6):841–848.

73. Kwon, Ki-Young; Wong, Kin L.; Pawin, Greg et. al. "Unidirectional Adsorbate Motion on a High-Symmetry Surface: "Walking" Molecules Can Stay the Course, Phys. Rev. Lett. 95, 166101 (2005) [Issue 16–14 October 2005]

Index

Printing and Binding: Stürtz GmbH, Würzburg